Love Shine

&

No F*cks To Give

A Guide to Embracing
Your Inner Light through Yoga

S.G. Bloomfield

Copyright © 2023 by S.G. Bloomfield

All rights reserved. No part of this publication may be reproduced, distributed, or transmitted in any form or by any means, including photocopying, recording, or other electronic or mechanical methods, without the prior written permission of the publisher, except in the case of brief quotations embodied in critical reviews and certain other non-commercial uses permitted by copyright law.

First Edition: 2023

Design and layout by Stefania Grieco

Published by Stefania Grieco

E-book ISBN: 978-1-7390129-6-0

Paperback ISBN: 978-1-7390129-4-6

Hardcover ISBN: 978-1-7390129-5-3

Important Note

Dear Reader,

Before we jump into our enlightening journey, here's a crucial nugget: I'm not a doctor. Although I'm an ardent writer and researcher, I lack the medical expertise you'd find in a healthcare professional.

Hence, always consult your doctor before applying anything you learn from this book to your routine. They're the right ones to guide you safely.

Remember, your body has its unique language, signaling you through discomfort or pain. So, listen keenly and respect these signals. Prioritize your health and well-being above all.

Let's explore together, but safety first!

S.G Bloomfield

In Gratitude and Love

For the place that first welcomed me into the warm embrace of yoga, the One Love One Heart Yoga Studio, nestled in the heart of Beeton, Ontario, Canada, this book is lovingly dedicated.

To the guiding spirit and relentless force behind our cherished sanctuary, the ever-inspiring owner whose vision breathed life into the place that transformed my journey forever, this one is for you.

And to the extraordinary ensemble of teachers, whose wisdom and patience unspooled the magic of yoga, stitch by stitch, until it became the fabric of my life. Your teachings have given me more than just poses and breathwork; they have given me a philosophy to live by, a community to belong to.

To the fellow students, the vibrant souls who shared the sacred space of the studio, laughter ringing in the air, sweat gleaming on our foreheads, and peace enveloping our hearts. Your journeys intertwined with mine, giving me the strength to persist, to evolve.

Our paths crossed in the comforting labyrinth of this yoga studio, each interaction, each lesson enriching my life in ways I could never have anticipated. Without these experiences, this book wouldn't have been possible.

So, with all my heart, this book is dedicated to you, the family I found in the tranquil corners of the One Love One Heart Yoga Studio. May the lessons we learned together resonate within these pages and extend beyond, touching lives, as you all have touched mine

.

CONTENTS

1 The Power of Love, Shine, and No F*cks to Give: Embracing Your Inner Light..........1

2 Love: Connecting with Yourself and Others through Yoga................................1

3 Shine: Unleashing Your Potential with Yoga...19

4 The Power of Breath in Yoga Practice 37

5 Embracing Fearlessness: Overcoming Fear and Judgment in Life....................57

6 Embracing Your Inner Shine: Discovering Your Unique Gifts and Talents.................77

7 Yoga for Emotional Healing: Nurturing Your Inner Self through Yoga 97

8 Yoga Philosophy for Cultivating Inner Light (Part 1).......................................115

9 Yoga Philosophy for Cultivating Inner Light (Part 2).......................................131

10 Honoring Your Inner Wisdom -..151

11 Owning Your Power..171

12 Beyond the Mat...193

13 Overcoming Obstacles on Your Yoga Adventure...211

14 Cultivating Compassion through Yoga..227

15 The Power of Ritual in Yoga...241

16 Yoga and Creativity: Unleashing Your Creative Potential..............................257

17 Exploring Yoga Styles and Traditions..271

18 Yoga Workshops, Retreats, and Teacher Training 289

19 Building a Supportive Yoga Community 309

20 Celebrating Your Inner Light: A Journey of Self-Discovery and Transformation ... 327

21 Yoga as a Lifestyle: Integrating Yoga Principles into Everyday Life 343

Love Shine and No F*cks To Give

A Guide to Embracing Your Inner Light through Yoga

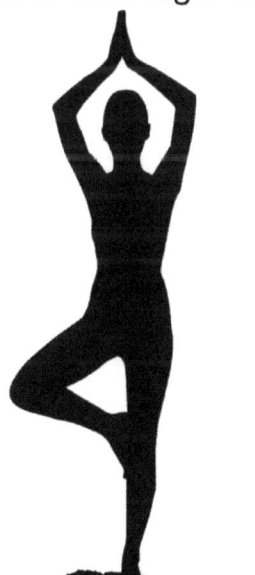

By S.G. Bloomfield

1

The Power of Love, Shine, and No F*cks to Give: Embracing Your Inner Light

Welcome to the World of Love, Shine, and No F*cks to Give

Imagine with me for a moment, you're on the verge of a vibrant exploration, a delightful expedition into the enchanting realm of love, luminosity, and unabashed self-expression. Picture yourself opening the first page of this book, "Love, Shine, and No F*cks to Give: A Guide to Embracing Your Inner Light through Yoga," and as you read each word, you start to feel the first stirrings of a hidden treasure within you - your unique happiness. Through the transformative practice of yoga, you will learn to nurture an internal state of bliss and cultivate an aura of radiance that knows no bounds.

The Challenges

In the bustling cacophony of today's world, we are often inundated with messages that seek to dictate our appearance, actions, and thoughts. Amidst this chaos, embracing your unique inner light and living an authentic life can seem like a Herculean task. No need to worry, dear traveler! This book is right here to guide you on your quest to unravel the mysteries of self-awareness, self-love, and inner tranquility. Yoga, a holistic practice that surpasses mere physicality, is the key that will unlock the door to this magical world.

The Journey and its Challenges

The path to self-discovery is a winding one, riddled with obstacles such as doubt, frustration, and discomfort. Yet, these challenges are an essential part of the voyage, serving to shape and refine your character as you traverse the road to enlightenment. Whether you're a seasoned yogi or a fledgling explorer just dipping your toes into the boundless ocean of yoga, this book will be your trusty compass, guiding you through the diverse and captivating landscape of a practice that has the power to unite you with your authentic self, nurture a sense of balance, and foster self-love and self-awareness.

As we kick off this exciting escapade together, we'll dig into the multifaceted world of yoga. We'll explore its physical aspects, like asana, as well as its more intangible elements, including meditation and mindfulness. Moreover, we will uncover the potent magic of love, gratitude, and self-appreciation as catalysts for elevating your overall happiness. By the time you reach the final pages of this book, you will possess a profound comprehension of your inner light and the tools required to embrace it with open arms.

Visualize us, stepping into this adventure together, kindling that dormant spark within and immersing ourselves in a life overflowing with love, brilliance, and bold authenticity. Doesn't that sound like an adventure worth taking?

So, come hither, my fellow explorers! Let's join forces in this exceptional quest for self-discovery and self-love.

As we start this extraordinary quest, you'll learn about the roots and history of yoga - a timeless ancient practice that has traveled across cultures, continents, and belief systems. We will examine the foundational principles of yoga philosophy, such as the eight limbs of yoga, which serve as a roadmap to guide you on your path to inner peace and self-realization.

Personal Anecdotes and Experiences

Throughout our journey, I'll share stories of my own playful exploration and experimentation with different yoga styles and approaches. My hope is that my experiences will inspire you to venture out, try new things, and find which styles resonate with your unique spirit. From the dynamic energy of Vinyasa to the serene stillness of Yin

Yoga, each style offers a distinctive experience, a new opportunity to connect with your innermost self.

Breathwork

As you delve deeper into the world of yoga, you will become intimately acquainted with the art of breathwork, or pranayama. Through a lighthearted exploration of various breathing techniques, you will unlock the power of your breath to soothe your mind, nourish your body, and ignite your inner light.

Meditation and Mindfulness

Alongside the physical practices of yoga, we will immerse ourselves in the calming embrace of meditation and mindfulness. As we playfully navigate the vast and tranquil realms of inner stillness, you will discover the immense power these practices hold in cultivating a sense of peace, harmony, and equanimity within your daily life.

Our delightful expedition will also illuminate the transformative potential of embracing love, gratitude, and self-appreciation. Through heartwarming anecdotes, enchanting exercises, and captivating stories, we will delve into the enchanting world of self-love and its capacity to elevate your overall well-being and sense of fulfillment.

Throughout our adventure, we'll meet a delightful bunch of wise and whimsical characters. Each one brings their unique insights and perspectives on the magical realms of love, shine, and no-holds-barred self-expression. Their delightful tales will serve as a source of inspiration, guiding you to new heights of self-discovery and personal growth.

As we traverse the enchanting landscape of yoga, we will encounter a multitude of delightful and thought-provoking activities, designed to spark your curiosity, ignite your creativity, and immerse you in the boundless joy of self-exploration. From whimsical journaling prompts to lighthearted movement exercises, these engaging activities will serve as stepping stones on your path to uncovering the hidden treasures of happiness nestled within your own being.

Together, we will explore the vibrant world of chakras, the subtle energy centers that govern our physical, emotional, and spiritual well-being. Through playful activities and enchanting visualizations, we will learn to balance and harmonize these vital energy centers, fostering a profound sense of equilibrium and glow that knows no bounds.

As our fun journey unfolds, we'll uncover the secrets of mantras - those sacred sounds and words that can lift us up, empower us, and light up our inner selves. Through the enchanting melodies of these mystical incantations, you will be transported to realms of boundless love, luminosity, and inner peace.

As we journey further into the mesmerizing world of yoga, we will delve into the captivating realms of Ayurveda, the ancient Indian science of life and wellness. Through a delightful exploration of its principles, you will discover how to cultivate a harmonious and vibrant existence, attuned to the rhythms of nature and your own unique constitution.

Our spirited adventure will also lead us to the gates of the enchanting world of mudras, the sacred hand gestures that hold the power to unlock the mysteries of the universe and awaken our dormant inner light. Through a lighthearted exploration of these mystical symbols, we will learn to harness their transformative potential, empowering us to step fully into our authentic selves.

As we approach the culmination of our extraordinary escapade, we will immerse ourselves in the art of ritual and celebration, learning to infuse our daily lives with an aura of joy, reverence, and gratitude. Through the creation of personal ceremonies and the sacred act of honoring life's milestones, we will discover the magic of embracing our inner light and sharing it with the world.

Finally, as we reach the concluding chapters of this book, you will gain a profound understanding of your internal glow and the tools required to embrace it wholeheartedly. As we bid farewell to our enchanting odyssey, you will be equipped with a treasure trove of knowledge, practices, and insights that will serve you well on your continued journey through the radiant realms of love, luminosity, and unabashed self-expression.

Invitation to the Journey

Now, step this way, my fellow adventurers! Let us embark on this remarkable voyage of self-discovery and self-affection. Hand in hand, we shall awaken our dormant potential and immerse ourselves in a life brimming with love, brilliance, and unapologetic authenticity.

Welcome, dear reader, to the delightful expedition that awaits you in the pages of "Love, Shine, and No F*cks to Give: A Guide to Embracing Your

The Power of Yoga for Self-Discovery and Embracing Your Inner Light

I still remember when I first discovered yoga, this ancient practice with a rich history. It felt like I had stumbled upon a tool, a key really, that unlocked a door to self-discovery. It was as if I was given an opportunity to connect deeply with my inner self and uncover my true essence. Through the physical postures, we develop a stronger connection with our bodies, becoming more sensitive to the various sensations that arise. This heightened awareness leads to a deeper understanding of our emotions and thoughts.

By bringing us into the present moment, yoga gently prompts us to let go of distractions and focus on our breath. This mindful presence cultivates greater awareness of our thoughts and emotions, helping us recognize patterns that may have limited our growth. In practicing yoga, we learn to observe ourselves without judgment, fostering self-awareness.

Furthermore, yoga enables us to develop compassion towards ourselves and others. As our understanding of our thoughts and emotions grows, we learn to accept ourselves and others more fully. This nurtures the foundations of self love and understanding, essential elements in the journey of self-discovery.

Think of this book as your travel buddy - always bright, cheerful, and supportive. And yoga? That's our sturdy ship, navigating us through the vast ocean of your inner world. Get ready to embark on an enjoyable adventure that celebrates humor and grace while making the profound wisdom of yoga accessible to everyone, whether you're an experienced yogi or a curious beginner. Together, let's begin this incredible journey to awaken our inner light and bask in the warmth of love, radiance, and unapologetic authenticity.

Dance with Your Inner Light: Yoga as a Tool for Joyful Self-Expression

Imagine a spark of joy, a flicker of creativity, a flame of authenticity - all these burning within us. That's our inner light waiting to dance in the open. Yoga, a versatile practice, offers a delightful avenue for self-expression and personal growth. By engaging in various light-hearted and playful yoga sequences, we can rediscover our inner child and bring a sense of wonder and curiosity into our daily lives. This extensive guide will provide an in-depth exploration of different yoga practices that can help us embrace our inner light more effectively.

Part 1: Laughter Yoga – A Joyful Journey to Inner Light

1.1. Understanding Laughter Yoga

Ever thought of yoga as a laughter riot? That's exactly what Laughter Yoga is - a fascinating mix of deep yogic breathing, laughter exercises, and gentle stretches that fill you with joy and tickles your funny bone. By consciously laughing and sharing it with others, we create an environment of lightheartedness and camaraderie.

1.2. Benefits of Laughter Yoga

Laughter Yoga offers numerous benefits, including:

1.2.1. Mood enhancement: Laughter releases endorphins, which are the body's natural feel-good chemicals. These endorphins can elevate our mood, making us feel happier and more relaxed.

1.2.2. Stress reduction: Laughter Yoga can help reduce stress by decreasing the levels of stress hormones like cortisol and adrenaline in the body. This promotes relaxation and improves overall mental health.

1.2.3. Immune system support: Regular laughter has been shown to strengthen the immune system, helping to protect us from illnesses and improve our overall health.

1.2.4. Creativity boost: Laughter Yoga can stimulate our creativity by encouraging us to think more freely and take ourselves less seriously.

1.2.5. Social connection: Laughter Yoga helps us bond with others, fostering a sense of community and belonging.

1.3. Starting Your Laughter Yoga Journey

To begin your Laughter Yoga journey, consider joining a local Laughter Yoga club or exploring online resources to find laughter exercises you can practice at home.

Part 2: Yoga and Creative Movement – Unlocking Your Inner Radiance

2.1. The Role of Creative Movement in Yoga:

What if your yoga mat became your dance floor, and every pose was a move that let your inner light shine? That's the magic of blending yoga with creative movement. These practices encourage us to let go of inhibitions, allowing our authentic selves to shine.

2.2. Creative Movement Practices to Explore

Discover the following creative movement practices:

2.2.1. Dance-inspired yoga: Dance-inspired yoga classes blend the elegance of dance with the grounding nature of yoga. These classes often integrate ballet, jazz, or contemporary dance movements with traditional yoga postures for a fun and invigorating experience. Seek out a local studio offering these classes or find online resources to guide your practice.

2.2.2. Yoga with music: Create a playlist of your favorite uplifting songs and flow through a yoga sequence in tune with the music. Let the rhythm inspire your movements, encouraging self-expression and creativity.

2.2.3. Freeform movement: Dedicate a portion of your practice to freeform movement, allowing your body to move spontaneously without any predetermined plan. This can help release any emotional or energetic blockages and foster a sense of freedom.

2.2.4. Partner yoga: Practice yoga with a friend or loved one, encouraging communication, trust, and connection. Partner yoga can deepen your practice, help you explore new poses, and foster a sense of playfulness.

Conclusion: Embracing the Inner Light Through Diverse Yoga Practices

By exploring and incorporating diverse yoga practices, such as Laughter Yoga and creative movement, we can effectively connect with our inner vitality, bolstering our well-being, creativity, and self-expression. These practices help us cultivate a deeper connection with ourselves, others, and the world around us. As we continue to nurture this inner vitality, we become more resilient, joyful, and true to ourselves in our daily lives.

Part 3: Yoga Nidra – Journey Into the Depths of the Subconscious

3.1. Understanding Yoga Nidra

Yoga Nidra, often called the 'yogic sleep,' is like a guided tour into the deepest corners of your subconscious mind while you relax and simply listen. This practice can help you gain insight into your innermost thoughts, desires, and emotions, fostering personal growth and self-awareness.

3.2. Benefits of Yoga Nidra

Yoga Nidra offers numerous benefits, including:

3.2.1. Deep relaxation: Yoga Nidra helps to calm the nervous system, promoting physical and mental relaxation.

3.2.2. Stress reduction: By relaxing the body and mind, Yoga Nidra can help alleviate stress and anxiety.

3.2.3. Improved sleep: Regular practice of Yoga Nidra can improve sleep quality and help address insomnia.

3.2.4. Emotional healing: Yoga Nidra can help release emotional blockages and support the healing of past traumas.

3.2.5. Enhanced creativity: By accessing the subconscious mind, Yoga Nidra can stimulate creative thinking and problem-solving abilities.

3.3. Incorporating Yoga Nidra Into Your Practice

To incorporate Yoga Nidra into your routine, consider attending a guided class or using recorded Yoga Nidra sessions available online. Set aside a quiet space and a dedicated time to practice this powerful meditation technique regularly.

Part 4: Kundalini Yoga – Awakening the Serpent Power

4.1. Understanding Kundalini Yoga

Imagine stirring up a dormant energy coiled at the base of your spine and letting it surge upwards. That's Kundalini Yoga for you - a blend of breathwork, meditation, and physical postures that awakens this transformative power within you. This energy, when awakened, travels up the spine, activating the chakras and expanding consciousness.

Years ago, before I began my journey into yoga, I found myself struggling with stress and a sense of disconnection. I was working in a high-pressure job, and the constant demands left me feeling drained, both physically and emotionally. I knew I needed a change, but I didn't know where to start.

Then, one evening, a friend invited me to a Kundalini Yoga class. I was hesitant at first - I had tried yoga once or twice before, but it had never really resonated with me. However, I decided to give it a chance.

The class was unlike anything I had experienced before. As we moved through the dynamic exercises and breathwork, I felt an energy awaken within me. It was like a spark had been ignited at the base of my spine, and as the class progressed, this energy began to rise, activating each chakra as it ascended. By the end of the class, I was left with a sense of tranquility and clarity I hadn't felt in years.

But it wasn't just the immediate effects of the practice that struck me. In the days following the class, I noticed a shift in my perspective. I was more aware of my thoughts and emotions, and I felt a renewed sense of connection with myself and the world around me. It was as if the Kundalini energy had illuminated a path towards self-discovery and personal growth.

That first Kundalini Yoga class marked the beginning of my yoga journey. It taught me that yoga is more than just a physical practice - it's a holistic approach to well-being, fostering physical health, emotional balance, self-awareness, and spiritual growth.

From there, I began to explore other yoga practices and techniques, each offering unique benefits and experiences. I discovered the joy of Laughter Yoga, the freedom of creative movement, the deep relaxation of Yoga Nidra, and the transformative power of breathwork. And with each new practice, I deepened my connection with my inner light, fostering resilience, joy, and authenticity in my daily life.

As I share these practices with you, I invite you to embark on your own journey of self-discovery and growth. Remember, the path to self-understanding and personal evolution is highly individual. Stay open to new experiences, honor your progress, and nurture your inner light. By embracing yoga in its many forms, you too can uncover your true potential and live a life of greater purpose, joy, and fulfillment.

4.2. Benefits of Kundalini Yoga

Kundalini Yoga offers numerous benefits, including:

4.2.1. Increased energy: By activating the Kundalini energy, this practice helps to boost vitality and stamina.

4.2.2. Expanded consciousness: Kundalini Yoga encourages spiritual growth and self-awareness, leading to a deeper understanding of oneself and the world.

4.2.3. Emotional balance: This practice helps to balance and harmonize the emotions, fostering mental stability and resilience.

4.2.4. Enhanced intuition: Regular practice of Kundalini Yoga can sharpen intuition and strengthen the connection to the inner guidance system.

4.2.5. Physical health: The dynamic movements and breathwork in Kundalini Yoga can improve strength, flexibility, and overall physical well-being.

4.3. Starting Your Kundalini Yoga Journey

To begin your Kundalini Yoga journey, seek out a qualified teacher or attend a local class to learn the proper techniques and guidance for this powerful practice. Online resources and books can also provide valuable information for those looking to explore Kundalini Yoga further. Kundalini Yoga is just one of many diverse practices that can help you connect with your inner light.

Discovering Your Inner Light Through Diverse Yoga Practices

As we dive into the world of Laughter Yoga, dance with creative movement, journey inward with Yoga Nidra, and awaken our power with Kundalini Yoga, we're essentially inviting our inner essence to fully express itself, promoting personal growth, self-expression, and spiritual development. As our connection to this inner glow deepens, we grow more resilient, joyful, and genuine in every aspect of our lives, illuminating the world around us and inspiring others on their journey of self-discovery and growth.

There are numerous yoga styles and techniques to explore, each offering unique benefits and experiences. The journey towards self-understanding and personal evolution is highly individual, so it's crucial to stay open to new experiences while seeking the path that resonates personally.

As you develop your yoga practice, focus on fostering a deeper connection with yourself, others, and the world. This connection will serve as a foundation for personal evolution, well-being, and fulfillment in all life aspects.

Here are suggestions for further exploration and deepening your yoga practice:

1. **Experiment with various yoga styles:** Discover the style that best suits your needs and preferences by trying different techniques, broadening your understanding of yoga's multifaceted world.
2. **Attend workshops and retreats:** Deepen your practice and connect with like-minded individuals by participating in yoga workshops and retreats.
3. **Read books and articles:** Expand your knowledge of yoga's philosophy, techniques, and benefits by immersing yourself in relevant literature.
4. **Connect with a community:** Join a local yoga studio, online group, or community center to share your journey and learn from fellow yoga enthusiasts.
5. **Be patient and compassionate with yourself:** Recognize that personal growth and self-discovery are ongoing processes, and approach your practice with curiosity and compassion.

Embarking on a journey of self-insight and personal development through yoga is a transformative experience. By exploring various practices, you can cultivate a profound connection with your inner light, fostering resilience, joy, and authenticity in daily life. As you nurture this inner radiance, you will not only grow personally but also inspire those around you on their own path of self-discovery and growth.

Deepening the Connection to Your Inner Light Through Mindfulness and Meditation

Yoga and meditation are intrinsically linked. As we deepen our yoga practice, we naturally cultivate mindfulness and presence. Through meditation, we can further enhance our self-awareness, connecting with our inner light in a more profound way.

Here are some meditation practices to complement your yoga journey:

- **Loving-kindness meditation (Metta):** Cultivate compassion for yourself and others by sending loving-kindness to yourself, loved ones, acquaintances, and even those you may find challenging. This meditation helps foster a sense of interconnectedness and warmth.
- **Body scan meditation:** Develop greater awareness of your body by systematically scanning your body from head to toe, observing any sensations that arise. This practice can help you become more attuned to your body's needs and foster a sense of self-care.
- **Mindfulness meditation:** Cultivate presence and acceptance by focusing on your breath or another anchor, such as the sensations in your body or the sounds around you. Gently redirect your attention to your anchor whenever your mind wanders.
- **Visualization:** Tap into your inner light by visualizing yourself as a radiant being, filled with love, joy, and compassion. Imagine this light expanding, enveloping your entire being, and extending outwards to touch the lives of those around you.

Journaling for Self-Discovery

Journaling can be an invaluable tool for self-discovery and self-expression. By recording your thoughts, feelings, and experiences, you can gain insight into your inner world, uncovering patterns and beliefs that shape your life.

Consider incorporating the following journaling prompts into your self-discovery journey:

- **Reflect on your yoga practice:** What did you notice about your body, mind, and emotions during your practice? What did you learn about yourself?
- **Gratitude:** Write down three things you're grateful for each day, fostering a sense of appreciation and abundance.
- **Dreams and aspirations:** Describe your ideal life and what steps you can take to bring your dreams to fruition. This can help clarify your desires and guide your actions.
- **Self-compassion:** Write a letter to yourself, offering compassion, understanding, and encouragement for any challenges you're facing.

Creating a Sacred Space for Self-Discovery

Designate a space in your home for your yoga and meditation practice, creating an environment that supports self-discovery, reflection, and inner growth. This space can serve as a sanctuary, where you can nurture your inner light and explore your authentic self.

Consider incorporating the following elements into your sacred space:

- A comfortable yoga mat or cushion for seated meditation
- Inspirational quotes, artwork, or objects that resonate with you
- Plants or flowers to create a sense of connection with nature
- Soft lighting, such as candles or fairy lights, to create a soothing atmosphere
- Aromatherapy, using essential oils or incense, to evoke a sense of calm and relaxation

Remember, your yoga practice and self-discovery journey are unique to you. Embrace your individuality, celebrate your progress, and honor your inner light. By nurturing self-awareness, compassion, and curiosity, you can uncover your true potential and live a life of greater purpose, joy, and fulfillment.

Cultivating Self-Awareness Through Breathwork

Breath serves as an essential gateway to self-awareness and self-regulation, offering a myriad of benefits and techniques. This brief introduction merely scratches the surface, as the fourth entire chapter delves deeper into the subject of breath. By cultivating a mindful connection to our breath, we can enrich our yoga practice, mitigate stress, and explore our emotional terrain. Consider integrating these breathwork techniques into your practice for optimal results:

1. **Ujjayi breath:** Also known as the "ocean breath," this technique involves constricting the back of the throat while inhaling and exhaling through the nose, creating a soothing, ocean-like sound. Ujjayi breath can help focus the mind and regulate the nervous system during your yoga practice.

2. **Nadi Shodhana (alternate nostril breathing):** This practice involves alternating between inhaling and exhaling through each nostril, helping to balance the energy in the body and promote mental clarity. Nadi Shodhana can be particularly beneficial before meditation or when seeking a sense of calm.

3. **Three-part breath (Dirgha Pranayama):** This technique involves breathing deeply into the belly, ribcage, and upper chest, promoting relaxation and stress relief. Practice three-part breath whenever you need to reconnect with your body and ground your energy.

While personal practices like breathwork are crucial, it's also important to remember we're part of a larger community.

Cultivating Connection Through Community

Strap in, my friend! The ride towards self-discovery? It's a wild one. Thrilling? Absolutely. A little tough sometimes? You bet. Connecting with a community of like-minded individuals can provide invaluable support, inspiration, and camaraderie. Consider the following ways to engage with your local yoga and wellness community:

Attend workshops, retreats, or festivals: Expand your horizons by participating in events that focus on personal growth, yoga, and holistic wellness. This can be a wonderful way to learn new skills, meet new people, and immerse yourself in a supportive environment.

Join local yoga or meditation groups: Seek out group classes, meetups, or online forums where you can share your experiences, ask questions, and offer encouragement to others on their journey.

Volunteer at a yoga studio or wellness center: Give back to your community by offering your time and talents. Volunteering can help you forge connections, develop new skills, and contribute to the growth and wellbeing of others.

In addition to connecting with a community, building a personal yoga library can further support your self-discovery journey.

Building a Personal Yoga Library

Imagine having a treasure trove of yoga and personal growth wisdom, right at your fingertips. Sounds great, doesn't it? That's the magic of building your very own yoga library.

Consider adding the following types of materials to your personal library:

- Books on yoga philosophy and history: Gain a deeper understanding of the origins and principles of yoga by exploring foundational texts such as the Yoga Sutras of Patanjali, the Bhagavad Gita, and the Hatha Yoga Pradipika.
- Instructional books and videos: Expand your knowledge of yoga asana, alignment, and sequencing with resources from experienced teachers and practitioners.
- Personal growth and self-help books: Explore a variety of topics related to self-discovery, mindfulness, and personal development to complement your yoga practice and support your inner journey.

What makes yoga your secret weapon for self-discovery and kindling your inner light? It's the trifecta of self-awareness, presence, and compassion that it brings to the table.

By engaging in a regular practice, exploring various techniques, and connecting with a supportive community, you can embark on a transformative journey that illuminates your authentic self and reveals the limitless potential within. Remember to be patient with yourself, honor your unique path, and celebrate the unfolding of your inner light.

Now that you understand the power of yoga for self-discovery and inner light, it's time to put it into practice with a simple 5-minute morning yoga routine.

Before we begin, I'd like to share a brief personal anecdote. Just a year ago, I found myself stressed and overwhelmed, juggling multiple responsibilities. One morning, I stumbled upon this exact 5-minute yoga routine, unsure of its impact. I decided to give it a try, and the transformation was remarkable. Starting the day with Banana Pose, I could feel the tension melting away. Windshield Wipers with an Easy Twist brought a sense of calm and focus, and Happy Baby Pose left me feeling joyful, just like its name suggests. Now, this routine has become an integral part of my mornings, infusing my day with positivity and energy. The best part? It only takes 5 minutes, a small investment for a day filled with peace and productivity.

5-Minute Morning Yoga Routine

Ready to kickstart your day with a simple 5-minute yoga routine? This is your golden ticket to a day brimming with personal growth and fresh, exciting possibilities.

This sequence is perfect for those who want to start their day on a positive note, or those who want to end it feeling relaxed and rejuvenated. We'll begin with Banana Pose, followed by Windshield Wipers with an Easy Twist, and concluding with Happy Baby Pose. Are you ready? Let's go!

Please remember to listen to your body and only perform these poses to your personal comfort and ability levels to avoid injury.

Banana Pose: Lie flat on your back, stretch your arms up and over your head, and reach your toes towards the end of the bed or mat. Take a deep breath in, and as you exhale, let your body sink into the bed or mat. Hold this pose for 3 deep breaths, and then slowly roll onto your right side, taking a quick pause.

Windshield Wipers with an Easy Twist: Bring both knees up towards your chest, and slowly drop them to the left side of your body. Take a deep breath in, and as you exhale, twist your torso to the right side, using your right hand to gently guide your left knee down towards the bed or mat. Hold this pose for 3 deep breaths, and then come back to center. Repeat on the other side, twisting towards the left side with your right knee dropped.

Happy Baby Pose: Bring both knees up towards your chest once more, and grab the outer edges of your feet with your hands. Open your knees wide, so that they're aligned with your armpits, and gently press your feet towards the ceiling as you pull down with your hands. This should create a gentle resistance that helps to open up your hips and lower back. Take deep breaths, and rock gently from side to side if it feels comfortable for you. Hold this pose for 3 deep breaths, and then slowly release your feet and lower your legs back down to the bed or mat.

Savasana (Corpse Pose): To close your morning practice, lie flat on your back, allowing your feet to fall open to either side and your arms to rest comfortably by your sides, palms facing upwards. Close your eyes, and take a few deep breaths, focusing on letting go of any tension in your body. Remain in Savasana for as long as you'd like, or until you feel ready to begin your day.

This quick and easy yoga routine is perfect for helping you connect with your inner light and setting the stage for personal growth and self-discovery throughout your day. As you continue to explore diverse yoga practices and deepen your connection to yourself and the world around you, remember to approach each new experience with an open heart and mind, ready to embrace the transformative power of yoga. By doing so, you will continue to grow and evolve, shining your inner light brightly and inspiring others to do the same.

As you move fluidly from one pose to another, picture yourself taking on the essence of Love Shine, spreading warmth and love with each stretch and twist, like you're the sun itself, casting its glow on everything around it. With each breath, let your heart open wide, allowing love to pour forth like a glorious, unstoppable waterfall. And just as the water cascades over every surface it touches, let your love envelop you and all those you encounter, shining bright and true.

Now, as you hold your poses and feel your muscles strengthen, channel that same unyielding spirit into embracing the philosophy of 'No F*cks to Give'. This isn't about being dismissive or uncaring, but about being true to yourself, unburdened by external judgments or unnecessary pressures. It's about living authentically, in line with your own truth and values. Stand tall in your own unique brilliance, like a majestic tree reaching for the sky, unapologetically taking up space, and extending its branches far and wide. With every playful sway and bend, remember that you, too, have the power to choose your own path, unburdened by the expectations or opinions of others.

So, as you continue with your day, carry the lessons of embracing self-love and standing firmly in your own authenticity, weaving these insights into the fabric of your being. With this newfound balance, you'll find that you can stand tall, radiate love, and let go of the trivial concerns that once weighed you down. Embrace this harmonious dance of self-love and authenticity, and let it guide you on a journey of self-discovery, growth, and boundless joy. This chapter has outlined the power of yoga for self-discovery and inner light, from yoga practices and meditation techniques to community engagement and building a personal yoga library. Carry these insights with you, as we delve deeper in the subsequent chapters, further illuminating your path towards self-discovery and personal growth.

2

Love: Connecting with Yourself and Others through Yoga

The role of self-love in yoga practice & Techniques for cultivating love in your practice

Let's embark together on a journey much like my own, where I found self-love, growth, and self-discovery through the ancient art of yoga. This chapter is your guide, drawn from my own experiences, on how yoga can cultivate self-awareness, love, and gratitude. With a playful spirit, we'll explore the transformative power of yoga and its beneficial effects on our well-being.

I recall a sunny morning when yoga entered my life, bringing peace, healing, and a refuge from anxiety and depression. As I stretched and strengthened, not only did my body become more flexible, but so did my mind, gaining clarity and tranquility. Through yoga, I learned about self-love and self-compassion, and how to accept my imperfections and limitations. Now, I feel more balanced and self-aware, even if I make mistakes sometimes.

Yoga has woven itself into the tapestry of my life, and the anticipation of its continued journey excites me. I invite you to join me on this transformative path. Close your eyes and take a deep breath, letting go of stress and tension.

Through yoga, I've discovered the power of self-love and the impact it has on my practice and well-being. It hasn't always been an easy journey, and along the way, I've found strategies to keep me centered and focused on self-love. Drawing from my experiences, I'd like to share some simple tips that helped me sprinkle self-love into my yoga practice and cultivate it in my life.

- **Set a guiding star:** Before I start each practice, I establish an intention that will guide my journey. This might be nurturing self-acceptance or releasing negative thoughts. This little ritual has been transformative for me. For example, you might say to yourself, "Today, I will practice self-compassion and let go of my judgments," or "I will focus on accepting my body as it is and embrace its uniqueness."
- **Practice self-compassion:** Treat yourself kindly during your practice, and remember that it's about growth, not perfection. When you stumble or find a pose challenging, avoid negative self-talk or criticism. Instead, offer yourself encouraging words, such as "It's okay, I'm learning and growing," or "I'm proud of myself for trying."
- **Connect with your breath:** Focus on your breath to quiet your mind and connect with yourself. As you inhale, imagine drawing in positive energy and love, and as you exhale, let go of any tension or negativity.
- **Practice gratitude:** At the end of your practice, be grateful for your body, mind, and spirit, and the progress you've made. Spend a few moments reflecting on the aspects of your practice or your life that you're thankful for, like the strength and flexibility you've gained or the mental clarity you've achieved.
- **Celebrate your accomplishments:** Acknowledge and celebrate your achievements, big or small. After a successful session, take a moment to recognize your progress, whether it's mastering a new pose or simply feeling more connected to your body and breath.

Try heart-opening poses, such as the Camel Pose, or practice Loving-Kindness meditation to further develop love and compassion in your practice. Remember that nurturing love goes beyond your yoga mat and involves how you treat yourself and others.

Yoga has many physical benefits that can help you feel more energetic and healthy. As you practice yoga, you'll notice your body becoming stronger, more flexible, and balanced. You don't need to be an expert to enjoy these benefits; even beginners can try poses like the downward-facing dog or the sun salutation to feel energized and refreshed.

Yoga also helps improve mental well-being by promoting relaxation and clarity. So, try practicing yoga in the morning to start your day with energy and enthusiasm. Embrace the power of yoga, and See your life evolve as you master each yoga pose.

With simple practices and dedication, you can grow love in your yoga practice and life. Breathe deeply, place your hand on your heart, and let love guide you. One significant way that I discovered self-love was through understanding and appreciating the physical benefits of yoga. Let's delve into that now.

Understanding the Physical Benefits of Yoga

Picture this: I used to welcome the dawn with a sigh, feeling as if the globe's weight had settled on my shoulders. Yoga became my antidote. You dread the long day ahead, and even the thought of leaving the warm cocoon of your bed seems like an impossible feat. We've all faced such mornings, haven't we? But what if I let you in on a secret? A simple practice that can turn your day around, infusing you with energy, clarity, and the enthusiasm to face anything that comes your way. The secret lies in the age-old practice of yoga, with its astonishing physical benefits.

Yoga, a practice that dates back thousands of years, is a remarkable tool for physical, mental, and spiritual well-being. As you incorporate yoga into your daily routine, you'll notice a transformation in your body, mind, and overall perspective on life. You'll feel stronger, more flexible, and more balanced. Your stress levels will dip, and you'll find yourself at ease, better equipped to handle life's challenges. And, as a bonus, you'll experience a deeper sense of inner peace and contentment.

The beauty of yoga is that you don't need to be an expert to reap its benefits. Even if you've never tried it before, there are simple poses that cater to all levels of experience and can help you feel the difference in your body and mind. Let's take a closer look at the benefits that yoga can provide. We'll break them down into categories for easier understanding: Physical Strength and Flexibility Benefits, Benefits Related to Circulation and Body Systems, Benefits Connected to Mental Well-being and Stress Reduction, and Benefits Related to Weight Management.

Physical strength and flexibility benefits:

1. **Enhanced flexibility:** I still remember the first time I attempted the Forward Fold (Uttanasana) and Pigeon Pose (Eka Pada Rajakapotasana). It was a struggle at first, but with consistency, I noticed my muscles and connective tissues started to stretch and give way. The stiffness that I once felt every morning began to fade away, replaced by a greater range of motion that made every movement feel more effortless.
2. **Improved muscle strength:** Yoga helps build and tone muscles, making you stronger and more resilient. Poses like Plank Pose (Kumbhakasana) and Chair Pose (Utkatasana) specifically target muscle strength.
3. **Better posture:** Yoga can help counteract poor posture by encouraging proper alignment of the spine and strengthening the muscles that support good posture. Poses such as Mountain Pose (Tadasana) and Cobra Pose (Bhujangasana) can be particularly beneficial.
4. **Enhanced balance:** The practice of yoga involves various poses like Tree Pose (Vrksasana) and Warrior III (Virabhadrasana III) that challenge your balance and stability.
5. **Increased stamina and endurance:** As you progress in your yoga practice, you'll find yourself able to hold poses like Boat Pose (Navasana) and Dolphin Plank Pose (Makara Adho Mukha Svanasana) for longer periods of time and move through more challenging sequences.
6. **Improved bone health:** Weight-bearing poses in yoga, such as Downward-Facing Dog (Adho Mukha Svanasana) and Triangle Pose (Trikonasana), can help strengthen your bones, reducing the risk of osteoporosis and other bone-related health issues. Moreover, the

flexibility and balance gained through yoga practice can help prevent falls and fractures, particularly in older adults.

7. **Reduced pain and inflammation:** Yoga has been shown to help alleviate chronic pain and inflammation. The physical strength and flexibility benefits we've just discussed play a pivotal role not only in our physical health but also contribute to self-love, confidence, and mental well-being. With these benefits, we're better equipped to embrace our bodies and minds in their entirety.

Having explored how yoga enhances our physical strength and flexibility, let's delve into how it optimizes our circulation and various body systems.

8. **Better circulation:** Yoga promotes healthy circulation by encouraging deep breathing and a variety of movements that stimulate blood flow. Poses like Legs-Up-The-Wall (Viparita Karani) and Seated Forward Bend (Paschimottanasana) can be particularly helpful.

9. **Improved respiratory function:** By focusing on deep, controlled breathing in poses like Bridge Pose (Setu Bandha Sarvangasana) and Lion's Breath (Simhasana), you'll strengthen your respiratory muscles, improve lung capacity, and enhance your overall respiratory function.

10. **Enhanced immune function:** The practice of yoga can help boost your immune system by reducing stress, promoting better sleep, and encouraging overall wellness. A stronger immune system can help protect you from illness and improve your ability to recover from injuries or health issues.

11. **Enhanced digestion:** Many yoga poses, like Supine Twist (Supta Matsyendrasana) and Wind-Relieving Pose (Pavanamuktasana), involve twisting and bending, which can help stimulate your digestive system and promote healthy bowel movements. Improved digestion can lead to increased nutrient absorption, reduced bloating, and overall better gut health.

Beyond the body, yoga also weaves its magic on our minds. Let's examine how it fosters mental well-being and aids in stress reduction.

12. **Reduced stress and anxiety:** Yoga's emphasis on mindfulness and relaxation can help lower stress levels and reduce anxiety. Poses like Child's Pose (Balasana) and Legs-Up-The-Wall Pose (Viparita Karani) promote a sense of calm and well-being, making it easier to cope with life's challenges. The deep breathing exercises and gentle movements in these poses can help you feel more at ease.
13. **Greater body awareness:** As you progress in your yoga practice, you'll become more in tune with your body, its needs, and its limitations. Poses like Tree Pose (Vrksasana) and Warrior II (Virabhadrasana II) can help you build balance and stability while fostering a strong connection to your body. This increased body awareness can help you make healthier choices, listen to your body's signals, and prevent injuries in other physical activities.
14. **Boosted energy levels:** The combination of deep breathing, mindful movement, and relaxation techniques in yoga can help increase your energy levels. Poses like Sun Salutations (Surya Namaskar) and Cobra Pose (Bhujangasana) can help you feel more alert and focused throughout the day, making it easier to tackle your daily tasks with enthusiasm.

Finally, one cannot ignore the role of yoga in maintaining a healthy weight. Let's consider how this ancient practice contributes to effective weight management.

15. **Weight management:** While yoga may not be as calorie-torching as some other forms of exercise, it can still play a role in weight management. Poses like Plank Pose (Kumbhakasana) and Chair Pose (Utkatasana) can help increase muscle mass, boost metabolism, and promote mindfulness, which can lead to healthier eating habits and better weight control.

As you can see, yoga offers an array of physical benefits that can have a profound impact on your overall health and well-being. By incorporating yoga into your daily routine, you can experience increased energy, improved mood, and a greater sense of balance and harmony in your life. Poses like the Tree pose (Vrksasana) and the Warrior pose (Virabhadrasana) can help improve your balance and focus, while the Downward-

Facing Dog pose (Adho Mukha Svanasana) and the Cobra pose (Bhujangasana) can enhance flexibility and strengthen the back.

So, the next time you find yourself facing a difficult morning or feeling overwhelmed, consider rolling out your yoga mat and allowing yourself the gift of movement, breath, and self-care. You might just find that yoga holds the key to unlocking a more vibrant, healthier, and happier you. So, embrace the beauty of the practice, and witness your life evolving, one pose at a time.

So, as we've journeyed together through the benefits and transformative power of yoga, remember that the true essence of yoga isn't about achieving the perfect pose but about cultivating self-love, self-acceptance, and growth. Whether it's improving physical strength, enhancing mental well-being, or fostering self-love, each pose and breath in yoga has the power to transform us.

Embrace yoga, embark on this transformative journey, and watch as each breath, each pose, nurtures your growth and blossoming.

But what does this journey of self-discovery entail? It involves cultivating awareness and mindfulness, which allow us to connect more deeply with ourselves and our experiences. With yoga as our guide, we can navigate the whirlwind of life with greater calm and clarity.

Cultivating Awareness and Mindfulness

Remember how we talked about embracing yoga for a vibrant, healthier, and happier you? Now, let's take it a step further.

Ever found yourself caught up in the whirlwind of life, where stress and anxiety are your constant companions? You're not alone. We've all been there. But imagine if there was a way to reconnect with our true selves, to bring back that lost balance. That's exactly where yoga, paired with mindfulness and awareness, comes into play.

Yoga serves as a foundation for developing mindfulness, as it brings together the body, mind, and breath in a harmonious and focused way. The physical postures, or asanas, encourage a deep connection with the body, while the breathwork, or pranayama, helps anchor the mind in the present moment. Integrating mindfulness techniques into your yoga practice can enhance the overall experience and benefits by fostering greater self-awareness, stress reduction, and mental clarity.

Let me share a bit of my journey with you. You know, there was a time when I was just like you, hustling through my days as an executive administrator. Then, I stumbled upon yoga, and boy, did it turn my life around! With each pose and breath, I was letting go of my worries and fears, and embracing the present. And the effect? I found myself more focused and efficient at work, while also being more patient and understanding with my family.

Experiencing the transformative power of yoga and mindfulness is hard to convey in words. In essence, it helped me become a more playful, graceful, and grateful person. If you're struggling with stress or seeking inner peace, I encourage you to give it a try. You may discover your own path to harmony and balance.

Ever dreamed of losing yourself in the moment? Picture this: You're standing at the edge of an endless ocean, with waves whispering secrets as they kiss the shore. The air smells like adventure, and the sun warms your skin, making you aware of the world's beauty and generosity. Right there, in that moment, you're one with the world, truly present and soaking it all in.

This is the power of mindfulness and cultivating awareness. By practicing a few simple techniques, you can harness this power for yourself:

1. Start your day with a brief meditation, focusing on your breath and bodily sensations. Try a body scan meditation, moving your attention from the top of your head to the tips of your toes, noticing any tension or sensations in each body part.
2. Immerse yourself in nature, paying close attention to the sights, sounds, and smells around you. Try a walking meditation, mindfully placing one foot in front of the other and observing the sensation of your feet touching the ground.
3. Practice simple yoga poses, like mountain pose or seated forward bend, to connect with your body and cultivate mindfulness. As you move through each pose, focus on your breath and the sensations in your body. Integrating mindfulness techniques, such as concentrating on the sensation of your feet grounding into the earth and your body swaying like a tree in the wind during tree pose, can deepen your connection to the present moment and enhance the overall experience.

4. Incorporate mindfulness into your daily activities, such as eating, cleaning, or brushing your teeth. For instance, when eating, savor each bite, noticing the flavors, textures, and sensations as you chew and swallow.

Remember, cultivating mindfulness and awareness takes time and practice. There will be moments when you feel distracted or overwhelmed. However, with patience and dedication, you can develop the skills needed to stay present and connected with the world around you.

Inhale deeply, let go of your worries and distractions, and embrace life's beauty and abundance. By practicing mindfulness and awareness in tandem with your yoga practice, you can truly experience the world in all its glory and live each moment to the fullest.

As you develop mindfulness and awareness through yoga, you may also notice an increased appreciation for life's beauty and the benefits of gratitude and self-love. These elements, when combined with yoga, create a powerful and uplifting experience.

Now that we've discussed the foundation of mindfulness, let's delve into how this practice can improve our interpersonal relationships and communication.

Mindfulness in Relationships and Communication

As we deepen our mindfulness practice, we can begin to notice the positive impact it has on our relationships and communication across various settings, such as work, family, or social situations. The ability to be present and attentive to others is an invaluable skill that can strengthen connections and enhance our interactions.

When we engage in mindful communication, we listen more intently and respond with empathy and understanding. By being fully present during conversations, we can grasp the emotions and intentions behind the words of others, leading to more meaningful connections and deeper relationships.

Here are some practical techniques that you can use to practice mindfulness in your relationships and communication:

1. Make a conscious effort to be present during conversations. For instance, at work meetings, turn off or silence your phone and close

irrelevant tabs on your computer, directing your focus to the speaker and the discussion at hand.

2. Practice active listening. This means not only hearing the words but also interpreting the emotions and intentions behind them. At a family gathering, ask open-ended questions like, "How did that experience make you feel?" to encourage your loved ones to share more and demonstrate your genuine interest.

3. Be aware of your body language. Maintain eye contact, nod in agreement, and lean slightly toward the person speaking during social events. These non-verbal cues signal that you're engaged and attentive.

4. Cultivate empathy and compassion. Put yourself in the speaker's shoes, attempting to understand their perspective and emotions. For example, if a colleague shares a challenging experience, try imagining how you would feel in a similar situation. This allows you to respond with kindness and compassion, even if you disagree.

5. Practice mindful speech. Be aware of your words, tone, and intent, ensuring that your message is clear, respectful, and honest. In a disagreement with a friend, choose language that expresses your feelings without blame or accusation, such as, "I felt hurt when you said that," to create a safe space for open and authentic communication.

As you incorporate mindfulness into your relationships and communication across various settings, you'll likely notice a newfound sense of understanding and harmony among your loved ones, colleagues, and friends.

Having discussed the impact of mindfulness on our relationships, let's now explore another important aspect of our yoga journey: gratitude and self-love.

Embracing Gratitude and Self-Love

Ready to take the next step on your yoga journey? Just as mindfulness can deepen your yoga practice, so too can gratitude and self-love. These practices can help you to further connect with your body, calm your mind, and open your heart. Ever thought about the transformative power of a simple 'thank you'? That's what gratitude can do. It can touch the coldest hearts and light them up. And when you weave this magical power of gratitude into your yoga practice, what you get is a beautiful tapestry of self-love and upliftment.

Imagine starting each day by acknowledging the amazing things around you: the warm sunlight on your face, the smile of a friend, or the comfort of a hot cup of tea. With gratitude, you can fill your days with positivity and kindness.

Yoga is more than a physical exercise; it's a way to learn about yourself, find inner peace, and discover the love and appreciation within you. By integrating gratitude into your yoga practice, you can enhance your overall well-being.

Begin by laying out your yoga mat and entering a space for self-reflection. As you move through poses like Anjaneyasana (Low Lunge) for embracing self-love, Balasana (Child's Pose) for surrendering to gratitude, or Vrksasana (Tree Pose) to cultivate inner balance and appreciation, let your thoughts wander through the good things in your life, savoring feelings of gratitude.

The power of gratitude isn't limited to yoga. It's a flexible practice that can be incorporated throughout your day. Pause to take a deep, refreshing breath, allowing the present moment to envelop you. Be kind to others, regardless of the size of the act, and notice how your heart swells with love and appreciation for the world.

Practicing gratitude isn't about ignoring life's challenges. Instead, it's about using appreciation as a tool to give you the strength to overcome obstacles and savor the beauty of the present moment.

With a playful attitude, step onto your yoga mat, open your heart, and let the remarkable blend of gratitude and self-love lift you up. Together, we'll navigate life's intricate tapestry, weaving gratitude, mindfulness, and awareness into every step.

The Ripple Effect of Mindfulness and Awareness

In my own journey, I've discovered that the practice of mindfulness and awareness extends far beyond our personal lives. When we consciously nurture presence and attentiveness, we can create a positive ripple effect that touches the lives of those around us.

Our thoughts, emotions, and actions all have consequences, and by practicing mindfulness, we can ensure that these consequences are positive and nurturing.

Consider the impact of small acts of kindness, like a warm smile, a comforting hug, or a simple word of encouragement. These gestures, though seemingly insignificant, can have a profound effect on someone's day. When we are mindful, we become more attuned to the needs and emotions of others, allowing us to respond with empathy and compassion.

In addition, by practicing mindfulness, we can reduce our own stress and anxiety, leading to a more balanced and peaceful life. This inner tranquility will naturally radiate outward, positively influencing the people around us. In turn, they may be inspired to cultivate their own mindfulness practice, creating a ripple effect of awareness and compassion throughout our communities.

Let me share a little story about how you can nurture the ripple effect of mindfulness and awareness in your daily life. Think of it as a personal guide to adding more kindness and consciousness into your everyday routine:

Practice random acts of kindness. Offer a helping hand, share a smile, or give someone a heartfelt compliment. These small gestures can have a lasting impact.

Be conscious of your environmental footprint. Mindfulness extends to our relationship with the planet. Take steps to reduce waste, conserve energy, and support sustainable practices.

Volunteer your time and talents. Offer your skills and resources to organizations and causes you're passionate about. This not only benefits others but also fosters personal growth and fulfillment.

Encourage mindfulness and awareness in others. Share your experiences and insights with friends and family, inspiring them to explore their own mindfulness journey.

By embracing mindfulness and awareness, we foster love, compassion, and understanding across the globe. Together, we work towards building a world where peace and harmony prevail.

Have you ever tried cultivating awareness and mindfulness through practices like yoga, meditation, and gratitude? Let me tell you, it's a life-changing journey that can bring about profound transformation. As we learn to be present and attentive, we can experience increased clarity, focus, and emotional balance. These qualities, in turn, can improve our mental and emotional well-being, enhance our relationships, and inspire positive change in the world around us.

The benefits of mindfulness are far-reaching, touching every aspect of our lives. From strengthening our physical health to promoting emotional resilience, mindfulness offers a pathway to personal growth and self-discovery.

As we become more attuned to our thoughts, emotions, and sensations, we can develop a deeper understanding of ourselves and the world around us.

By weaving gratitude, mindfulness, and awareness into every step of our journey, we can nurture an inner sanctuary of peace and tranquility. This inner calm will serve as a foundation for personal transformation, allowing us to approach life's challenges with grace, resilience, and wisdom.

As we continue to deepen our mindfulness practice, we can experience a sense of interconnectedness with all living beings, cultivating empathy, compassion, and kindness. This interconnectedness can inspire us to take action, catalyzing positive change that extends far beyond our personal lives.

In a world that can often feel chaotic and uncertain, mindfulness offers a guiding light, illuminating a path towards wholeness, healing, and harmony. By embracing the practices of awareness and mindfulness, we can embark on a journey that leads not only to personal fulfillment but also to the collective well-being of our global community.

So, as you venture forth on your path of mindfulness and awareness, remember that every step, every breath, and every moment of presence contributes to the intricate tapestry of life. Embrace the journey, and let the transformative power of mindfulness light the way.

As part of this journey, let's take a moment to explore a practical application of mindfulness and awareness: a gentle yoga practice. This practice is not only a means to strengthen the body but also a powerful tool to cultivate the mental and emotional benefits of mindfulness.

Gentle 15-minute Practice to Cultivate Gratitude and Self-Love

Welcome to this 15-minute level 1 yoga sequence focused on cultivating gratitude and self-love. This gentle practice is perfect for beginners and those with no previous yoga experience. Please remember to listen to your body and modify the poses as needed. Let's get started!

1. Easy Pose (Sukhasana)
   - Sit on your mat or a cushion with your legs crossed and hands resting on your knees.
   - Close your eyes, lengthen your spine, and take a few deep breaths to set your intention for gratitude and self-love.

[Modification: If sitting cross-legged is uncomfortable, extend your legs in front of you or place a cushion under your hips.]

2. Seated Side Stretch
   - Inhale, and as you exhale, reach your left hand to the right side of your mat, stretching the left side of your body.
   - Hold for 3 breaths, then return to the center and repeat on the right side.

[Modification: If the stretch is too intense, reduce the reach of your hand or bend your elbow.]

3. Cat-Cow Pose (Marjaryasana-Bitilasana)
   - Transition onto your hands and knees with your wrists under your shoulders and knees under your hips.
   - Inhale as you arch your back and lift your chest and tailbone towards the ceiling (Cow pose).
   - Exhale as you round your back and tuck your chin towards your chest (Cat pose).

[Modification: If your wrists hurt, you can make fists or use yoga blocks under your hands.]

4. Child's Pose (Balasana)

- Sit back onto your heels, spread your knees apart, and extend your arms out in front of you, resting your forehead on the mat.
- Take deep breaths, holding this position for 2 minutes.

[Modification: If it's hard to sit back on your heels, place a cushion or folded blanket between your hips and heels.]

5. Downward-Facing Dog (Adho Mukha Svanasana)
   - From Child's pose, tuck your toes under and lift your hips up and back, straightening your legs and pressing your heels towards the ground.
   - Hold for 5 breaths.

[Modification: If this pose is challenging, bend your knees slightly and keep your heels lifted off the floor.]

6. Standing Forward Fold (Uttanasana)
   - From Downward-facing dog, walk your feet towards your hands and let your upper body hang, bending your knees if necessary.
   - Hold for 5 breaths.

[Modification: If it's hard to reach the ground, bend your knees or use yoga blocks under your hands.]

7. Mountain Pose (Tadasana)
   - Slowly roll up to a standing position, stacking your vertebrae one at a time.
   - Stand tall, feet hip-width apart, your weight distributed evenly across both feet.
   - Hold for 5 breaths.

[Modification: If standing for extended periods is uncomfortable, use a wall for support.]

8. Tree Pose (Vrksasana)
   - Shift your weight onto your left foot, and place your right foot on your left ankle, calf, or inner thigh.
   - Bring your hands together in front of your heart, and hold for 5 breaths.

[Modification: If balance is a challenge, keep your toes on the ground and heel against your ankle.]

9. Seated Twist (Ardha Matsyendrasana)
   - Sit down on your mat with both legs extended in front of you.
   - Bend your right knee, placing your right foot outside your left thigh.
   - As you inhale, lift your left arm, and as you exhale, twist your torso to the right.
   - Place your left elbow on the outside of your right knee and your right hand behind you for support.
   - Look over your right shoulder, keeping your spine tall.
   - Hold for 5 breaths, then switch sides.

[Modification: If the twist is too intense, keep your left hand on your right knee and your right hand on the floor behind you.]

10. Corpse Pose (Savasana)
    - Lay down on your back and let your legs fall open.
    - Let your arms relax at your sides, palms facing upwards.
    - Close your eyes, breathe deeply, and relax your entire body into the mat.
    - Stay here for 5 minutes or as long as you need.

[Modification: If you have lower back discomfort, place a folded blanket or bolster under your knees.]

This yoga sequence is designed to promote feelings of gratitude and self-love. Remember to move with your breath and listen to your body, making modifications as needed. Let the practice serve you and support your intention of cultivating gratitude and self-love.

To finish your practice, gently wiggle your fingers and toes, then stretch your arms overhead and take a deep breath. Slowly roll to one side, using your arms to push yourself up to a comfortable seated position.

Bring your hands together at your heart, and bow your head, acknowledging the gratitude and self-love you've cultivated throughout this practice.

Namaste.

As you move through the rest of your day, remember the feelings of gratitude and self-love that you've experienced during this yoga practice. Carry these feelings with you and share them with others to create a more loving and compassionate world. Thank you for joining me in this 15-minute level 1 yoga sequence.

As we draw this chapter to a close, I want you to pause for a moment. Take a deep breath and truly feel the transformative power of the level 1 yoga sequence we've journeyed through together. Can you feel that energy buzzing in your fingertips? That's the power of mindfulness and yoga.

As we delve into the next chapter, "Shine: Unleashing Your Potential with Yoga," we'll explore advanced techniques and practices that will take you even further on your journey toward self-discovery and personal growth.

The light within you is boundless, and with each mindful breath and movement, it shines brighter. So, take a deep breath, and prepare to unlock the full potential of your inner light in our next chapter.

The light that yoga sheds on life is something special. It is transformative. It does not just change the way we see things; it transforms the person who sees.

~ B.K.S. Iyengar ~

3
Shine: Unleashing Your Potential with Yoga

As we step into Chapter 3, "Shine: Unleashing Your Potential with Yoga," let me share with you a personal story of transformation that showcases the true magic of yoga.

Imagine being a young soul grappling with social anxiety and depression. Now picture this: yoga comes into the picture, wrapping you in a warm, gentle embrace that instills a newfound sense of self-assurance and bravery to face your fears.

As they delved deeper into this practice, they discovered an innate ability to connect with others, and social situations became less daunting. Their overall mental well-being flourished, and their mood lifted.

Through continuous dedication to yoga, the author grew more balanced and resilient, now confidently navigating life's challenges. The transformative potential of yoga lies in its capacity to foster personal growth, healing, and self-discovery by embracing one's uniqueness. As you embark on your own yoga journey, remember to cultivate your practice at your own pace. Before long, you too will have an inspiring story to share, reflecting the power of yoga in your life.

Tapping into your inner strength and potential

You know how we, as humans, often stumble upon roadblocks in our minds and bodies, leaving us feeling trapped and riddled with self-doubt?

Overcoming these constraints can be difficult, but yoga provides a comprehensive means to connect with our body, mind, and spirit, revealing hidden strengths and capabilities. More than just physical exercise, yoga includes breathwork, meditation, and mindfulness, working in harmony to help us uncover the power and potential within us, achieve mental clarity, heighten bodily awareness, and establish a profound connection with our true selves.

Yoga aids us in tapping into our inner strength and potential in several ways. Firstly, it enhances physical strength and flexibility, which subsequently boosts confidence and self-awareness. As we challenge ourselves with new poses and movements, we conquer physical obstacles and recognize our true strength.

Moreover, yoga fosters mindfulness and awareness, crucial factors for unlocking our full potential. By quieting our minds and focusing on the present moment, we become more receptive to our thoughts and emotions, allowing for better self-understanding and insight into our inner workings. This heightened awareness helps us detect negative patterns or beliefs that may impede our progress, enabling us to address them and advance with greater confidence and clarity.

Dipping your toes into the world of yoga might seem a bit daunting, especially if you're new to it, but let's break it down together, shall we?

Fear not, as the following sections will delve into specific ways to achieve this through yoga, introducing beginner-friendly poses and practices to help you start your journey with ease. Incorporating simple breathing exercises, gentle stretches, and easy-to-follow poses, a solid foundation can be built, fostering growth and development over time for those new to yoga.

If you seek to access your inner strength and potential, consider incorporating yoga into your life. Its holistic approach and emphasis on mindfulness and self-awareness could be the key to unlocking your true potential and realizing your full capabilities.

Letting Go of Comparison and Judgment

In this digital age we're living in, it's so easy to get caught up in the swirl of 'perfection' we see everywhere, right? This often involves measuring ourselves against others on social media, friends, family members, and even our past selves. We might criticize our bodies, abilities, and self-worth. However, practicing yoga and embodying its principles, such as

"Ahimsa," can help us find inner peace and self-acceptance by freeing ourselves from these tendencies.

Yoga, an ancient practice with a rich history, has helped countless individuals achieve tranquility, balance, and harmony. It encourages us to release our inclination to compare and judge, focusing on the present moment and self-acceptance.

Ahimsa, a core principle of yoga, represents non-violence, including not only avoiding harm to others but also cultivating self-compassion and kindness. Practicing Ahimsa fosters gentleness, understanding, and self-acceptance, embracing our flaws.

As we relinquish comparison and judgment, we can fully experience yoga's transformative power. We become attuned to our unique strengths and weaknesses, promoting personal growth tailored to individual needs. This self-awareness leads to self-love and appreciation, which extends to our relationships and interactions.

By letting go of judgment and adopting Ahimsa, we unlock yoga's full potential, nurturing self-love and generating positive ripple effects throughout every aspect of our lives.

Developing a Personal Yoga Practice

Crafting your own yoga practice is like creating a personalized road map to self-growth and discovery, taking into account all the unique twists and turns that make you, you. Begin by setting clear intentions, such as finding inner peace or improving physical strength, which will serve as a guiding force throughout your practice. Explore various yoga styles like Hatha, Vinyasa, or Yin and seek guidance from experienced practitioners through classes, online tutorials, or books to find a style that resonates with you. Establishing a consistent routine, whether daily or weekly, is essential for personal growth and development. Create a comfortable, distraction-free space filled with positive energy to cultivate tranquility and focus during your practice. Lastly, remember to listen to your body, modifying or skipping poses as needed, and practice self-compassion.

1. **Set clear intentions:** Begin your practice by setting an intention, whether it be finding inner peace, cultivating gratitude, or improving your physical strength. This intention will serve as a guiding force throughout your practice, helping you stay focused and motivated.

2. **Explore styles and seek guidance:** Find your preferred style by exploring different styles of yoga, such as Hatha, Vinyasa, or Yin, and don't be afraid to seek guidance from experienced practitioners, whether it be through attending a class, watching online tutorials, or reading books on yoga. This will provide you with valuable insights, support, and help you find a style that resonates with you.

3. **Establish a routine:** Dedicate a specific time each day or week for your practice, whether it be in the morning or evening, and commit to maintaining this schedule. Consistency is key for personal growth and development.

4. **Create a comfortable space:** Set up a designated space for your practice, free from distractions and filled with positive energy. This will help you cultivate a sense of tranquility and focus during your practice.

5. **Listen to your body:** Remember to always be gentle with yourself and listen to your body's needs. If a pose feels uncomfortable or painful, modify or skip it altogether. It's essential to honor your body and practice self-compassion.

Through dedication and commitment, you will gradually unveil your true potential, allowing your inner light to shine brightly and guide you on your path to self-discovery and personal growth.

Your journey of personal growth and self-discovery, try incorporating easy yoga poses into your routine. These beginner-friendly postures will not only help you develop your physical abilities but also deepen your connection to your breath and inner self.

Easy Yoga Poses for Unleashing Your Potential

Ready to unlock your potential? Let's dive into these three transformative yoga postures that not only amp up your strength, flexibility, and balance, but also deepen your connection to your breath and inner self.

These poses promote physical, mental, and emotional growth, laying the foundation for a fulfilling, lifelong yoga experience. Explore the unique benefits of each posture and understand how they contribute to your personal development journey.

1. **Inversions: Legs-Up-The-Wall Pose (Viparita Karani):**

This restorative inversion pose allows you to relax and rejuvenate while promoting healthy circulation. Begin by placing a folded blanket or bolster near the wall. Sit down with your left or right side against the wall, and then gently lie down on your back. Slowly swing your legs up the wall as you pivot your body to face the ceiling. Ensure that your buttocks are resting on the blanket or bolster, and your lower back is supported. Place your arms alongside your body with your palms facing up, or rest your hands on your belly. Close your eyes and focus on taking slow, deep breaths as you hold the pose for 5-15 minutes. To release, gently bend your knees, roll to one side, and slowly come up to a seated position.

2. **Seated Twist (Ardha Matsyendrasana):**

Introduce gentle twists into your practice with this seated pose. Sit on your mat with your legs extended in front of you. Bend your right knee and place your right foot outside your left thigh. Bend your left knee and tuck your left foot near your right hip. Inhale to lengthen your spine, and exhale as you twist gently to the right, placing your right hand behind you and your left elbow on the outside of your right knee. Hold the twist for a few breaths, and then repeat on the other side.

3. **Bridge Pose (Setu Bandha Sarvangasana):**

Start exploring backbends with this accessible pose that helps to strengthen your back muscles and open your chest. Lie on your back with your knees bent and feet hip-width apart, close to your buttocks. Press your feet into the mat, and lift your hips toward the ceiling, while keeping your shoulders and head on the ground. You can interlace your fingers under your hips or place your palms flat on the mat for support.

Stay in the pose for a few breaths, then gently lower your hips back to the mat.

Having familiarized yourself with these three transformative yoga postures, you are now prepared to embark on a journey of self-exploration and personal growth. As you continue to practice and refine these poses, you'll not only enhance your physical abilities but also deepen your connection with your inner self. This newfound understanding will empower you to embrace your individuality, allowing you to tailor your yoga practice to your unique needs and aspirations, ultimately leading you to discover the multitude of benefits that extend far beyond the mat.

Embracing Your Individuality

Think about this - each time you step onto your yoga mat, you're about to embark on a truly personal journey, one that leads you beyond the physical and into a realm of self-discovery and personal growth. And guess what? The key to unlocking this journey is your individuality.

A key aspect of this journey is recognizing and embracing your individuality. The practice of yoga is not a one-size-fits-all approach; rather, it is a deeply personal and unique experience for each individual.

Getting to grips with the importance of your unique stamp on your yoga journey is like finding the compass to your personal growth. Each person comes to yoga with their own background, experiences, and personal goals. These factors contribute to the uniqueness of each individual's practice. It is important to remember that everyone's body is different, and as such, the practice of yoga will be distinct for each person. Comparing oneself to others can be counterproductive and may hinder the development of a meaningful and fulfilling practice.

Instead, focus on your own progress and celebrate the victories and breakthroughs you achieve along the way. It is crucial to listen to your body and to honor its limitations and strengths. This self-awareness will help you develop a practice that is tailor-made for your needs, allowing you to cultivate a deeper connection with your mind, body, and spirit.

As you embark on your yoga journey, remember to be patient and kind to yourself. Individual development and self-realization are ongoing processes, and it is natural to experience setbacks and challenges along the way. Embrace these moments as opportunities to learn and grow, and allow yourself the space to explore and adjust your practice as needed.

Get curious and adventurous. Try different styles of yoga, learn from various teachers, and explore diverse environments. You're on a quest to find what clicks with you the most. This exploration will help you cultivate a practice that feels authentic and nourishing to your individual needs. Remember, your yoga journey is your own, and it is important to honor and nurture your unique path.

The practice of yoga is a profoundly intimate voyage, where individuality plays a vital role. As you continue to explore and deepen your practice, remember to embrace your uniqueness and allow it to guide you on your path to self-discovery and personal growth. By honoring your individuality and adapting your practice to suit your needs, you will ultimately uncover the transformative power of yoga and experience the many benefits it has to offer.

Let's take a step back for a moment and remember, as we've been saying, yoga is like your personal odyssey - one that champions individuality and self-discovery. This journey is open to everyone, regardless of age, body type, or fitness level. Unfortunately, there are still many stereotypes and misconceptions surrounding yoga that may deter some from experiencing its transformative power. It's essential to dispel these myths and emphasize that yoga truly is for everyone.

One of the most common misconceptions about yoga is that it's only for the flexible or fit. This stereotype likely stems from images of experienced yogis bending their bodies into seemingly impossible positions. However, these images do not represent the entirety of the yoga practice. Yoga is a holistic practice that encompasses more than just physical flexibility – it also includes breath control, meditation, and ethical principles.

The truth is, yoga is for every body. There is no prerequisite level of flexibility or fitness required to begin a yoga practice. Yoga postures, or asanas, can be modified to accommodate different body types, physical limitations, and experience levels. Props such as blocks, straps, and bolsters can also be utilized to support the body and make poses more accessible. As you practice, you will naturally develop greater flexibility and strength, but these are not prerequisites for starting your journey.

Another misconception is that yoga is only for a specific age group, particularly the young. This couldn't be further from the truth. Yoga is an inclusive practice that can be adapted to meet the needs of individuals of all ages. There are various styles of yoga that cater to different levels of intensity and physical ability, such as gentle yoga, chair yoga, and restorative yoga, which are particularly suitable for older adults or those with limited mobility.

Furthermore, some people may assume that yoga is only for women. However, yoga is equally beneficial for men and women, offering physical, mental, and emotional benefits for all. Historically, yoga was predominantly practiced by men, and it has only been in more recent times that it has become associated with women. Today, more and more men are embracing yoga as a way to increase flexibility, build strength, and relieve stress.

It's crucial to challenge these stereotypes and ensure that everyone feels welcome and encouraged to explore the world of yoga. Regardless of your age, gender, body type, or fitness level, yoga offers an opportunity to connect with yourself, develop self-awareness, and cultivate inner peace. By embracing the inclusive nature of yoga, we can encourage more people to embark on their own personal journeys and discover the transformative power of this ancient practice.

To really get on board with the inclusive vibe of yoga, we need to give ourselves a big bear hug, imperfections and all. This means practicing self-compassion and self-acceptance, which are vital to personal growth and development. By letting go of self-judgment and expectations, we can create a supportive environment in which to learn from our mistakes and flourish.

Self-compassion is the ability to treat ourselves kindly, even when we feel that we have fallen short or made mistakes. In the context of yoga, this means recognizing that it's okay not to be perfect in every pose or to struggle with certain aspects of the practice. Yoga is not about achieving perfection; it's about connecting with our bodies, minds, and spirits in a meaningful way. By cultivating self-compassion, we can be patient with ourselves as we progress on our yoga journey, celebrating small victories along the way and recognizing that every step is valuable.

One effective way to practice self-compassion is to become aware of the negative thoughts that can arise during yoga practice. When these thoughts appear, gently remind yourself that it's normal to face challenges and that growth comes from overcoming them.

Replace self-critical thoughts with kind, supportive affirmations, such as, "I am doing my best," or "I am growing and learning."

Self-acceptance is another key component of embracing imperfection in yoga. This means acknowledging our strengths and limitations without judgment. By accepting ourselves as we are, we can let go of the need to measure our progress against unrealistic expectations or the accomplishments of others. Instead, we can focus on the unique path that lies before us, embracing the learning opportunities that come our way.

To cultivate self-acceptance, begin by setting realistic and attainable goals for your yoga practice. Focus on the aspects that resonate with you, and be open to adjusting your goals as you progress. Remember that yoga is a lifelong journey, and there is always room for growth and change.

As you practice yoga, keep in mind that mistakes are an essential part of the learning process. Instead of viewing them as failures, see them as opportunities to grow and refine your practice. When you stumble or struggle in a pose, take a deep breath, and remind yourself that this is a normal part of the journey. Allow yourself to be imperfect, and embrace the wisdom that arises from these experiences.

Embracing imperfection in yoga is crucial for fostering self-compassion and self-acceptance. By letting go of self-judgment and expectations, we can create a nurturing environment for individual development and self-exploration. Remember that yoga is a journey of self-exploration, and as we learn to be kinder and more accepting of ourselves, we inspire others to do the same, creating a more inclusive and compassionate yoga community for everyone.

The Power of Intention-Setting in Yoga: Cultivating Individuality

Remember when we chatted about the idea of setting an intention earlier? Let's revisit that. Though it may appear insignificant or unnecessary, setting an intention is actually a crucial step in enhancing your yoga experience. It works in harmony with two other key components: maintaining a steady breath and remaining present throughout your practice. Together, these three elements create a powerful foundation for a fulfilling and transformative yoga journey, even for those who are new to the practice.

As we delve deeper into the world of yoga, it becomes clear that this versatile and holistic practice goes beyond physical postures, offering numerous benefits to its practitioners. One crucial aspect of yoga that can help you truly personalize your practice is the power of intention-setting. By setting intentions, you can cultivate individuality and foster a deeper connection with yourself. Here, we will discuss the importance of setting intentions in your yoga practice and provide examples of intentions, such as self-love, inner peace, or mental clarity. Additionally, we will guide you on how to set your own intentions, making yoga an enriching and transformative experience for you.

Setting an intention is like turning the spotlight of your thoughts onto a particular purpose or goal. In the context of yoga, an intention is a guiding principle that aligns your practice with your innermost values and aspirations. Setting intentions allows you to create a customized experience that resonates with your unique needs and desires, thus promoting individuality.

There are various intentions that you can set for your yoga practice, depending on what you want to achieve or emphasize. Here are some examples:

- **Self-love:** Setting an intention of self-love encourages you to accept and cherish yourself unconditionally, nurturing a positive relationship with your body and mind. This intention can help you cultivate self-compassion, fostering a more loving and supportive inner dialogue.
- **Inner peace:** Choosing inner peace as your intention allows you to focus on calming your mind and releasing stress. As you move through your practice, you become more aware of your breath and the present moment, leading to a serene and tranquil state of being.
- **Mental clarity:** When your intention is mental clarity, your yoga practice becomes an opportunity to declutter your mind from distracting thoughts and emotions. This focus can help you improve concentration and attain a sharper, more attentive mental state.

Want to set your own intentions? Here's a step-by-step guide to make it easier for you:

- **Reflect:** Before starting your yoga practice, take a moment to reflect on your current state of mind and emotions. Identify areas in your life that require attention or improvement.

- **Choose your intention:** Based on your reflection, select an intention that resonates with your personal needs and aspirations. This intention should inspire and motivate you to commit to your practice.
- **Visualize:** Close your eyes and visualize your intention, imagining how it feels when it is fully embodied. Hold this image in your mind, allowing it to sink into your consciousness.
- **Incorporate into practice:** As you begin your yoga practice, keep your intention at the forefront of your mind. Allow it to guide your movements, breath, and focus throughout your session.
- **Revisit and revise:** Periodically reassess your intentions and adjust them as needed. This ensures that your yoga practice remains aligned with your evolving needs and goals.

Intention-setting is a powerful tool that can help you personalize your yoga practice and foster individuality. By setting intentions, such as self-love, inner peace, or mental clarity, you create a more meaningful and purpose-driven experience on the mat. So, the next time you roll out your yoga mat, take a moment to set an intention, and watch as it transforms your practice and your life.

As you embrace intention-setting in your yoga practice, you'll find that it opens up a new path to discovering your true self. This journey of self-discovery is crucial in helping you live a more authentic and fulfilling life. By fostering a deeper connection with your inner self through yoga, you unlock the gateway to self-discovery, and ultimately, a more genuine and satisfying existence. The transformative power of intention-setting not only enhances your time on the mat but also enables you to break free from the confines of a life that doesn't feel like your own. So, let's delve deeper into the concept of living authentically and uncover the secrets to achieving self-discovery and fulfillment.

Living Authentically – The Gateway to Self-Discovery and Fulfillment

Ever catch yourself in a moment, feeling like the life you're leading isn't quite yours? Like you've stumbled onto someone else's stage, playing a part that just doesn't feel right? If you do, you're not alone. Many people feel this way, and the reason is simple – they're not living authentically.

But what does it mean to live authentically? It means being true to yourself, your values, your needs, and your feelings. It means not compromising your integrity or pretending to be someone you're not. It means living your truth, even when it's hard.

There's a lot to be said for living authentically. For starters, it's a ticket to a heightened sense of self-awareness. When you're marching to the beat of your own drum, you start to tune in more deeply to your thoughts, feelings, and actions. You also become more aware of the impact you have on others and the world around you.

Living authentically also brings inner peace. When you're not trying to please others or meet their expectations, you can relax and be yourself. You no longer have to pretend or wear a mask. You can just be.

But living authentically is not always easy. It requires courage, self-awareness, and a strong connection to your inner guidance. That's why it's important to have practical tips and strategies to help you stay on track.

One of the golden rules of living authentically? Stay true to your values. These are the guiding stars in the constellation of your life, the things that really mean the world to you, like being honest, showing integrity, having compassion, and displaying respect. When you live in alignment with your values, you feel a sense of purpose and fulfillment.

Another way to live authentically is to set boundaries. Boundaries are the limits you set on what you're willing to accept from others. They help you protect your energy and your well-being. When you set boundaries, you communicate your needs and feelings honestly, which leads to better relationships.

Let me tell you, yoga can be a game-changer when it comes to living authentically. It's a bridge that connects you to your body, mind, and spirit, and it's a brilliant teacher, showing you how to listen to your inner guidance. Yoga also helps you cultivate self-awareness, which is essential for living authentically.

To use yoga to live more authentically, start by practicing self-reflection. Take some time to think about your values, your needs, and your feelings. Then, use your yoga practice to connect with your inner guidance. Pay attention to how your body feels, and listen to your intuition.

While you're on the mat, try to stay in the now and keep a non-judgmental mindset. Let go of any 'shoulds' or goals, and just allow yourself to be in the moment. This will help you nurture a sense of inner peace and authenticity.

Living authentically is not always easy, but it's worth it. When you live in alignment with your true self, you experience greater fulfillment, purpose, and joy. So, take the first step today. Connect with your inner guidance, stay true to your values, and live your truth. You won't regret it.

Yoga practices for living authentically

Picture this - waking up each morning with a sense of purpose and joy, feeling a deep connection to your true self, and brimming with confidence about your decisions. While achieving this level of authenticity can be challenging, there are enjoyable and practical exercises you can incorporate into your daily routine to help you live a more authentic life without any pressure or expectations.

But fear not, my friend! There are fun and practical exercises that you can incorporate into your daily routine to help you live a more authentic life. And the best part? You only have to do the ones that resonate with you. No pressure, no expectations, just the opportunity to try something new and potentially life-changing.

So let's dive in, shall we? First on our list is the "Gratitude Journal." Carve out a few moments each day to jot down three things you're grateful for. It could be anything - big or small, simple or complex, just something that brings a smile to your lips or a warm feeling in your heart. By focusing on the good in your life, you shift your perspective and attract more positivity into your daily experience.

Next, we have "Soulful Silence." Set aside five minutes each day to simply sit in silence. No music, no phone, no distractions. Just you and your thoughts. This is a powerful way to connect with your inner self, to listen to the whispers of your intuition, and to gain clarity on your desires and goals.

Moving on, we have "Random Acts of Kindness." This one is pretty self-explanatory, but it's important nonetheless. Do something kind for someone else each day. It can be as simple as holding the door open for someone or as grand as buying a stranger a cup of coffee. By focusing on giving, you not only brighten someone else's day but also create a ripple effect of positivity in your own life.

Last but not least, we have "Passionate Pursuits." Make time each week to do something that you're truly passionate about. Whether it's painting, writing, dancing, or hiking, engage in an activity that brings you joy and fulfillment. This is a powerful way to connect with your true self, to tap into your creativity and imagination, and to remind yourself of what makes you truly happy.

So there you have it, my friend. Fun and practical exercises to help you live a more authentic life. Remember, you only have to do the ones that resonate with you. If you're on the fence about one, try it out anyway. You never know, you might just discover something new about yourself and find yourself living a more joyful and fulfilling life.

10 Minute Hatha Practice

this 10-minute Hatha yoga practice designed for beginners, aimed at unleashing your potential. Remember to listen to your body, and feel free to use the modifications provided to deepen your practice.

1. Begin in Easy Pose (Sukhasana)
   - Sit on your mat with your legs crossed and hands resting on your knees.
   - Lengthen your spine, and take a few deep breaths to center yourself.
   - If you wish to go deeper, close your eyes and visualize your potential expanding with each breath.

[Modification: If your hips are tight, sit on a cushion or folded blanket to elevate your hips and create a more comfortable position.]

2. Seated Cat-Cow (Marjaryasana-Bitilasana)
   - Inhale, arch your back, and lift your chest and gaze upward.
   - Exhale, round your back, tuck your chin and engage your core.
   - Repeat for five breaths, syncing your movements with your breath.
3. Seated Forward Fold (Paschimottanasana)
   - Extend your legs in front of you, keeping your feet flexed.
   - Inhale and reach your arms overhead, lengthening your spine.

- Exhale, fold forward from your hips, reaching for your shins or feet.
- Hold for 5 breaths. To deepen, fold further and relax your neck and shoulders.

[Modification: If it is uncomfortable to do this pose seated, transition to a tabletop position to practice cat-cow pose.]

4. Transition to Tabletop Position
   - Place your hands under your shoulders and knees under your hips.
   - Spread your fingers wide and press into the mat for support.

[Modification: If your wrists are sensitive, balance on your fists or use yoga blocks under your hands. If your knees are uncomfortable, place a folded blanket underneath them for added cushion. If holding your weight on your shoulders is challenging, lower onto your forearms.]

5. Downward-Facing Dog (Adho Mukha Svanasana)
   - Tuck your toes, lift your hips, and straighten your legs.
   - Keep your knees slightly bent if needed, and lengthen your spine.
   - Hold for 5 breaths. To deepen, press your chest towards your thighs and your heels towards the ground.

[Modification: If this pose is challenging, bend your knees slightly and keep your heels lifted off the floor.]

6. Low Lunge (Anjaneyasana)
   - Low Lunge (Anjaneyasana)
   - Step your right foot forward between your hands.
   - Lower your left knee to the ground, keeping your right knee stacked over your ankle.
   - Inhale and lift your arms overhead, keeping your shoulders relaxed.
   - Hold for 3 breaths. To deepen, sink your hips further and arch your back. Repeat on the left side.

[Modification: If you experience knee discomfort, place a folded blanket under your back knee.]

7. Warrior II (Virabhadrasana II)

- From a standing position, step your left foot back and turn it out 90 degrees.
- Bend your right knee, stacking it over your ankle, and extend your arms out to the sides.
- Gaze over your right fingertips and hold for 3 breaths.
- To deepen, sink deeper into the lunge and engage your core.
- Repeat on the left side.

[Modification: If it is challenging to maintain balance in this pose, perform it near a wall, so you can touch the wall with your back hand for extra support.]

8. Tree Pose (Vrksasana)
   - Stand tall and shift your weight to your left foot.
   - Place your right foot on your left ankle, calf, or inner thigh (avoid the knee).
   - Bring your hands to your heart center or extend them overhead.
   - Hold for 5 breaths, focusing on your balance. To deepen, close your eyes.
   - Repeat on the right side.

[Modification: If balance is a challenge, rest your hand on a chair or wall for support.]

9. Child's Pose (Balasana)
   - Kneel on your mat, with your big toes touching and knees hip-width apart.
   - Sit back on your heels and fold forward, extending your arms in front of you.
   - Rest your forehead on the mat and breathe deeply for 5 breaths.
   - To deepen, bring your knees wider and extend your arms further.

[Modification: If your forehead doesn't comfortably reach the mat, place a yoga block or bolster under it for support.]

Here is a guided meditation designed to unleash your potential, allow yourself to embrace your true abilities and talents. As we begin, let's set the intention to cultivate a lighthearted and gracious atmosphere, filling our hearts with warmth, joy, and a sense of wonder.

being disturbed. Let yourself sink into the space, and gently close your eyes. Take a few deep breaths, inhaling through your nose and exhaling through your mouth. Feel your body relax as you sink into the present moment.

Now, bring your awareness to your heart center, envisioning a radiant, golden light emanating from within. This light represents your innate potential, waiting to be unlocked and shared with the world. As you breathe in, visualize this light growing brighter and more vibrant.

In your mind's eye, imagine a beautiful, lush garden filled with various types of plants, flowers, and trees. This garden represents the different aspects of your life and the many seeds of potential within you. Notice how the golden light from your heart is illuminating the garden, nurturing and encouraging growth.

Begin to walk through this garden of potential, observing the unique qualities of each plant and flower. As you continue to stroll, notice a path leading to a small, elegant fountain. Make your way towards it, feeling the light from your heart creating a warm and inviting atmosphere.

As you arrive at the fountain, take a moment to appreciate the delicate flow of water, symbolizing the continuous flow of life and the ever-present opportunities for growth. Gently cup your hands and gather some water, feeling its cool and refreshing touch.

Now, bring the water to the golden light emanating from your heart. As the water meets the light, watch as the brilliance intensifies, creating a luminous aura around you. Feel the energy of your potential expanding, reaching out to every corner of your being.

With this newfound energy, return to the garden, and as you walk amongst the plants and flowers, gently sprinkle the glowing water upon them. Observe as they instantly flourish and thrive, blossoming with newfound vigor and beauty. This represents the incredible power you hold within to manifest your dreams and aspirations.

As you continue to nurture the garden, remember that your potential is limitless, and every challenge or setback is simply an opportunity for growth. You have the power to create a life of abundance, love, and success, for you are the gardener of your own destiny.

Now, slowly bring your awareness back to your physical surroundings. Take a few deep, nourishing breaths, feeling a renewed sense of confidence and purpose. When you are ready, gently open your eyes, carrying with you the knowledge that your potential is boundless and waiting to be shared with the world.

Go forth, dear friend, and let your light shine brightly, for the world is truly a better place with your unique gifts and talents.

4

The Power of Breath in Yoga Practice

What if I told you that the secret to a healthier, happier life has been under your nose the whole time? That's right, my friend, the simple act of breathing, when done mindfully, can bring about amazing transformations in our lives.

Meet Emma, a yoga and pranayama practitioner. For years, she led a high-pressure, tension-filled life, until she discovered the transformative power of breathwork. Emma shares, 'Pranayama helped me find inner peace and balance in my hectic daily routine. I now have a deeper connection to my body, mind, and spirit.' Her tale testifies to the profound changes breathwork can bring.

Ready to unlock your potential and soar to new heights just by mastering your breath? Let's embark on this enlightening adventure into the world of breath work together, my friend, and witness its profound influence on our lives.

You'll hear real-life stories that highlight how breath work can enhance emotional well-being, physical health, athletic performance, and even help cope with PTSD. As we delve deeper into these narratives, you'll see the amazing power of breath work in transforming lives in various situations.

1. Mental Clarity and Emotional Balance:

Are you eager to discover how mental clarity and emotional balance, much like Catherine achieved, is within your reach?

Let's dive into the first transformative story

Catherine, a thriving 35-year-old entrepreneur, reached a pivotal moment in her life upon embracing breath work. As she juggled work and family life, her days became consumed by relentless stress and anxiety. Overwhelm frequently set in, placing a strain on her personal relationships. Serendipitously, her life took a transformative turn when she attended a breath work workshop. By regularly practicing alternate nostril breathing (Nadi Shodhana), Catherine reaped immense benefits. Incorporating this technique into her morning routine, during work breaks, and before bedtime, she successfully cultivated mental clarity and emotional balance.

Catherine's journey reveals the transformative power of breath work. It shows us that even in the midst of stress, it's possible to find balance.

Takeaway: Regular practice of alternate nostril breathing can bring about mental clarity and emotional balance, helping to manage stress effectively.

2. Physical Health and Overall Well-being:

Curious about how breath work could impact your physical health and overall well-being? Unveil Sophia's story:

Now, let's explore another tale of transformation. Meet Sophia.

Sophia, a devoted yoga enthusiast, grappled with persistent fatigue and a compromised immune system. In search of a remedy to bolster her health, she discovered the Wim Hof Method. Venturing through a variety of breath work techniques, including the Wim Hof Method, Sophia experienced significant improvements in sleep quality, heightened focus, and enhanced athletic performance, ultimately fostering her overall well-being. Her journey serves as a powerful testament to the profound influence of breath work on physical health and holistic wellness.

Sophia's experience demonstrates how breathwork can rejuvenate us physically. It's remarkable to think that feeling energized and healthy could be as simple as focusing on your breath!

Takeaway: Techniques like the Wim Hof Method can help boost sleep quality, focus, and athletic performance, contributing to overall well-being.

3. Athletic Performance:

Can breath work enhance athletic performance? Let's learn from James' story

Let's shift gears and explore athletics through James' journey.

At 50 years old, marathon runner James stumbled upon the benefits of breath work while recovering from a running injury. Frustrated by his inability to train, he searched for alternative methods to maintain both his physical fitness and mental resilience. That's when he discovered diaphragmatic breathing. Eagerly, James integrated this technique into his daily routine for relaxation purposes and to enhance his lung capacity. As a result, he experienced a marked improvement in stress levels and overall well-being. As his injury healed, he was pleasantly surprised to find his running performance had also improved. James' journey highlights the remarkable ways breath work can complement physical training and elevate athletic performance.

James' experience is a prime example of how breath work can actually boost our physical performance. Who knew breathing could be a game changer for athletes, right?

Takeaway: Diaphragmatic breathing can be a powerful tool to enhance lung capacity, reduce stress levels, and improve athletic performance.

4. Emotional Control and Coping with PTSD:

Can breath work serve as a solution for emotional control and coping with PTSD? Delve into Michael's story:

Our next story is a bit intense, but it's an important one. Are you ready to hear about Michael's journey?

Having served as a soldier and grappling with post-traumatic stress disorder (PTSD) upon his return from deployment, Michael found solace through the guidance of a therapist. Introducing him to the technique of box breathing, the therapist offered a means to manage his PTSD symptoms. Diligently employing this method, Michael practiced box breathing prior to and following triggering events, as well as amidst high-stress situations. This greatly enhanced his emotional regulation, positively affecting both his professional and social interactions. Gradually, Michael gained a stronger sense of control over his emotions, enabling him to better navigate life's challenges.

Michael's journey is a powerful one, showing how breath work can help us regain control during the most turbulent times. It's truly remarkable, don't you think?

Takeaway: Techniques like box breathing can significantly improve emotional regulation, especially for individuals coping with conditions like PTSD.

5. Stress Management and Enhanced Productivity:

Can breathwork enhance productivity and manage stress? Discover how Angela found solace:

Next, let's delve into the life of Angela, a graduate student who found a unique solution to her academic stress.

At 28 years old, Angela was a graduate student who sought solace in breath work amidst the taxing demands of academia. With relentless deadlines and towering expectations, her stress levels reached unprecedented heights. It was then that a friend introduced her to the practice of box breathing, which Angela began to incorporate during study breaks and anxiety-ridden moments. Through this straightforward technique, she was able to refocus her mind, soothe her racing thoughts, and reinvigorate her energy for her studies. Angela's journey serves as a testament to the adaptable nature of breath work in not only managing stress but also in bolstering productivity across various aspects of life.

Angela's story proves that even in the most stressful situations, breath work can be our ally. Imagine, being able to refocus and reenergize, just by breathing!

Takeaway: Even amidst high stress situations, box breathing can help refocus the mind and boost productivity.

The transformative power of breath work isn't exclusive to individuals like Catherine, Sophia, James, Michael, and Angela; many others, including the author of this book, have experienced its benefits. Let me share with you my journey. But before we dive into that, it's important to understand that breath work techniques have become globally recognized as valuable resources for personal growth and well-being.

Much like Catherine and the others, I too was once in a place where stress seemed like an insurmountable mountain. But breath work changed that for me. My mind raced incessantly, never granting me a moment of true tranquility. However, everything changed when I attended a transformative breath work group session led by an empathetic instructor. As we practiced various breathing exercises, I felt my anxiety dissipate, and a wave of calm washed over me.

Integrating breathwork into my daily routine had a profound impact on my lifestyle. My stress was significantly reduced, my attention at work became more acute, the frequency of my headaches diminished, and my sleep improved. Breath work taught me the virtues of patience and self-compassion, allowing me to accept my imperfections as part of my unique journey. I also found that integrating breath work into my morning routine set the tone for a clear and focused day, better equipping me to handle life's challenges.

For someone with no experience in yoga or breath work, this journey can be seen as an odyssey of self-discovery.

Through the power of mindful breathing, we can tap into a reservoir of healing and self-understanding. This inner tranquility equips us to navigate life's obstacles with grace and ease. As I continue to practice breath work, I find comfort in the sanctuary of my breath, realizing that I am part of a transformative, shared journey and not alone in this experience.

6. Self-Care and Overall Well-being:

How can breath work contribute to self-care and overall well-being? Examine Tina's story:

Let's wrap up our stories with Tina. Ready to hear how breath work changed her life?

Tina, a 42-year-old single mother, was searching for ways to cope with the demands of raising two children while working a full-time job. A colleague suggested exploring breath work as a way to balance her busy schedule and promote self-care. Tina started practicing the breath of fire (Kapalabhati) and found that it provided her with the energy boost she needed to get through her long days. Over time, Tina also noticed improvements in her digestive health, reduced stress levels, and increased mental clarity. Her story is an example of how breath work can be a powerful tool for self-care and overall well-being in even the busiest of lives.

Tina's story is so relatable, isn't it? Balancing work, kids, and self-care is a juggling act, but breath work seems to make it a little easier!

Breathwork has redefined my life, and it holds the same potential for anyone embarking on this journey, even those with no prior experience. Through its practices, I've found ways to alleviate stress, enhance my concentration, and discover a sense of inner peace. Incorporating these breathing exercises into my daily routine, I've experienced fewer headaches, improved sleep quality, and a newfound sense of patience and self-compassion. I've learned to embrace my imperfections as part of my unique journey. This transformative power of mindful breathing equips us to navigate life's obstacles with grace and ease. It's a shared journey towards healing and self-understanding that reminds us that we are not alone in this experience.

As time has passed, breath work techniques have evolved, spreading worldwide and becoming integral to diverse cultural practices. Nowadays, breath work is viewed as a valuable means of fostering personal growth, well-being, and self-enhancement.

If you're new to this world of yoga or breath work, don't worry, you're not alone. Starting this journey could be your ticket to self-discovery, healing, and inner peace. It's about tapping into your potential, finding that resilience to tackle life's hurdles, and seeking comfort in the sanctuary of your breath. As you continue practicing, you'll realize that this journey isn't a solitary one, but a shared experience of transformation.

Remember, the key to unlocking the full potential of breath work is consistency. Start by selecting one or two techniques that resonate with you, and commit to practicing them daily. As you become more comfortable, feel free to incorporate additional techniques or modify existing ones to suit your individual needs.

Consider breath work as a unique avenue for inward transformation. By integrating these techniques into a daily routine, one can unlock increased mental clarity, emotional stability, physical strength, and flexibility.

As evident from the stories of Catherine, Sophia, James, Michael, Angela, and even my own experience, breath work is a transformative tool for everyone. It's a journey that we undertake individually, yet it unites us in our shared experience of transformation and growth.

This empowering practice is available to all, regardless of yoga experience. Through dedicated practice, you can access numerous benefits, improving mental focus, emotional equilibrium, and physical abilities.

Breathing Techniques Explored

Allow me to guide you through a fundamental breath work technique that's been a game changer in my personal journey - Diaphragmatic Breathing, or simply, Belly Breathing. Imagine taking a deep, nourishing breath through your nose. Feel your diaphragm contract, your belly expand like a balloon. Now, let that breath out slowly through your mouth or nose, gently deflating. Simple, right? Incredibly effective, diaphragmatic breathing melts away stress and anxiety, ushering in a deep sense of relaxation and tranquility. It stimulates the part of the nervous system that helps us relax and digest, while calming the part that governs the stress response.

An Unexpected Path to Mindfulness

Just like many, I found it challenging to incorporate meditation and mindfulness into my life. But a simple breathing technique was the key to unlocking my potential. When work got stressful and I felt like I was losing balance, my friend Tina suggested trying the 4-7-8 breathing technique every morning for a week. Skeptical, I decided to give it a shot.

Before beginning any of the breathing techniques discussed in this chapter, it is essential to start with two fundamental steps that lay the foundation for an effective practice. Although these steps may not be explicitly mentioned in the instructions for each technique, please note that they apply to all of them:

- **Step 1:** Find a comfortable seated or lying position.

- **Step 2:** Place one hand on your chest and the other on your abdomen.

Once you've settled into a comfortable position, close your eyes and take a few deep breaths to center yourself. This preparation will help you achieve a more focused and effective practice as you explore the various techniques. Always remember to begin with these two steps to ensure optimal results from your breath work.

In my early days of practicing these techniques, I found it fascinating how such simple steps could make a big difference. It's like a secret key to a whole new world of calm and focus.

4-7-8 breathing technique

Step by step instructions on how to perform the technique:

- **Step 3:** Now that you're settled, draw a deep breath through your nose, let your abdomen rise as it fills with air.

- **Step 4:** Slowly release the breath through your mouth or nose, feel your abdomen fall.

- **Step 5:** Continue this for several breaths. Focus on each breath and the rise and fall of your abdomen.

Take your time with this technique, there's no rush. Remember, it's your journey.

In the beginning, it might feel a little odd or challenging, but don't worry, it's completely normal. I had the same experience when I first started, but with time and practice, it became second nature.

Alternate Nostril Breathing (Nadi Shodhana)

Another potent and transformative technique is alternate nostril breathing, known as Nadi Shodhana in Sanskrit. This method involves using the thumb and ring finger to alternate between closing off one nostril at a time, inhaling and exhaling in a slow, controlled manner. Nadi Shodhana is known to balance the left and right sides of the brain, promoting mental clarity, focus, and emotional balance.

Step by step instructions on how to perform alternate nostril breathing (Nadi Shodhana):

- **Step 3:** Having already completed Step 1 and Step 2, bring your right hand to your nose. Use your thumb to close your right nostril and your ring finger to close your left nostril.

- **Step 4:** Close your right nostril with your thumb and inhale slowly through your left nostril.

- **Step 5:** Close your left nostril with your ring finger and hold your breath briefly.

- **Step 6:** Release your thumb and exhale slowly through your right nostril.

- **Step 7:** Inhale through your right nostril, then close it with your thumb, and exhale through your left nostril.

- **Step 8:** Repeat this cycle for several rounds, focusing on the flow of your breath.

As you go through this, try to visualize the balance you're creating within your body.

Breath of Fire (Kapalabhati)

A more energizing technique is the breath of fire, or Kapalabhati. This practice involves rapid, forceful exhalations through the nose, with passive inhalations. Kapalabhati is believed to ignite the digestive system, supercharge energy levels, and purify the respiratory system, leaving you feeling refreshed and invigorated.

Step by step instructions on how to perform the breath of fire (Kapalabhati):

- **Step 3:** After completing Step 1 and Step 2 mentioned earlier, Take a deep breath in through your nose.

- **Step 4:** Forcefully exhale through your nose, contracting your abdominal muscles.

- **Step 5:** Allow your inhalation to be passive, as your abdomen naturally relaxes.

- **Step 6:** Continue this cycle of forceful exhalations and passive inhalations for 30 seconds to a minute, focusing on the rhythm of your breath.

Box Breathing (Four-Square Breathing)

Box breathing, or four-square breathing, is a simple yet effective technique to promote relaxation and focus. This method involves inhaling for four counts, holding the breath for four counts, exhaling for four counts, and holding the breath again for four counts.

Box breathing, a favorite among athletes and military personnel, is a go-to technique for managing stress and boosting performance under pressure.

Step by step instructions on how to perform box breathing (four-square breathing):

- **Step 3:** After completing Step 1 and Step 2 mentioned earlier, Inhale through your nose for a count of four.

- **Step 4:** Hold your breath for a count of four.

- **Step 5:** Exhale through your mouth or nose for a count of four.

- **Step 6:** Hold your breath again for a count of four.

- **Step 7:** Repeat this cycle for several rounds, focusing on the count and your breath.

Wim Hof Method

Lastly, let's explore the Wim Hof Method, a technique that combines deep breathing exercises with cold exposure. The Wim Hof Method involves taking 30 to 40 deep, rapid breaths, followed by a breath retention and a controlled exhale. This technique is said to improve the immune system, increase energy levels, and reduce inflammation.

Step by step instructions on how to perform the Wim Hof Method:

In addition to the breathing exercises, the Wim Hof Method also incorporates cold exposure. This can be achieved through activities like cold showers, ice baths, or swimming in cold water. The combination of deep breathing exercises and cold exposure is believed to provide the full range of benefits associated with the Wim Hof Method. If you're interested in incorporating cold exposure into your practice, make sure to research and follow appropriate safety guidelines.

Heads up! The Wim Hof Method can be quite intense. It's not for everyone, especially if you have certain medical conditions. Always check with your healthcare professional before giving this one a try.

- **Step 1:** As with the other techniques, begin by finding a comfortable seated or lying position, and place one hand on your chest and the other on your abdomen.

- **Step 2:** After completing Step 1, take 30 to 40 deep, rapid breaths, inhaling through your nose or mouth and exhaling through your mouth.

- **Step 3:** After the final breath, exhale fully and hold your breath for as long as you comfortably can.

- **Step 4:** Inhale deeply and hold your breath for 10 to 15 seconds.

- **Step 5:** Exhale and relax, allowing your breath to return to normal.

- **Step 6:** Repeat this cycle for two or three rounds, focusing on the rhythm of your breath.

Remember to consult with a healthcare professional before starting any new breath work practices, especially if you have any pre-existing medical conditions.

Breath work is transformative. By incorporating these techniques into your daily routine, you unlock potential. You achieve balance. You embrace mindfulness. You find fulfillment.

Embrace the power of breath and experience its positive impact on your mental, emotional, and physical health

Techniques for Cultivating Breath Awareness and Control

When you dive into yoga and pranayama, you're signing up for more than just physical strength and flexibility. You're stepping onto a path of personal growth and self-discovery. To make the most of your practice, incorporating interactive elements like exercises, self-assessments, and guided meditations can be highly beneficial. These elements will deepen your understanding of various concepts and techniques, making your experience more engaging and rewarding. By integrating these practices, you will empower yourself to apply the techniques in your own life and achieve balance, mindfulness, and fulfillment.

Breath awareness and control are fundamental aspects of yoga and pranayama practice. Developing these skills allows you to fully engage with your body, enhance your focus, and improve your overall well-being. To help you cultivate breath awareness and control, try the following exercises:

Three-Part Breath (or as it's traditionally known, Dirga Pranayama):

a. Settle down in a comfy spot, either sitting or lying down.

b. Gently close your eyes and take a handful of deep breaths to ground yourself.

c. Draw in a slow breath, filling your belly first, followed by your ribs, and finally let it reach your upper chest.

d. Gradually let go of the breath, first from your upper chest, then your ribs, and finally let your belly deflate.

e. Keep this three-section breathing going for a few rounds, staying in tune with the rhythm of your breath and the feeling of each part filling and emptying.

Really take the time to connect with each part of your body as you breathe. It's a journey of discovery, after all.

Pursed-Lip Breathing:

Helps control breathlessness Improves lung function

Step-by-step instructions:

a. Find a comfortable seated or lying position.

b. Inhale slowly through your nose, keeping your mouth closed.

c. Purse your lips as if you were going to whistle.

d. Exhale slowly through your pursed lips, taking twice as long to exhale as you did to inhale.

e. Repeat this cycle for several breaths, focusing on the rhythm of your breath and the sensation of your breath passing through your pursed lips.

Ujjayi Breathing (Ocean Breath):

Encourages relaxation Boosts concentration during yoga practice

Step-by-step instructions:

> a. Find a comfortable seated or lying position.
>
> b. Close your eyes and take a few deep breaths to center yourself.
>
> c. Inhale slowly and deeply through your nose, slightly constricting the back of your throat to create a soft, ocean-like sound.
>
> d. Exhale slowly and deeply through your nose, maintaining the constriction in your throat to continue the ocean-like sound.
>
> e. Repeat this cycle for several breaths, focusing on the sound of your breath and the sensation in your throat.

These breathing techniques offer various benefits for mental and physical well-being. Practicing them regularly can help manage stress, improve focus, and promote overall relaxation. Always remember to consult with a healthcare professional before trying any new breathing technique, especially if you have any pre-existing medical conditions.

Breath Visualization Exercise:

> a. Find a comfortable seated position.
>
> b. Close your eyes and take a few deep, slow breaths to center yourself.
>
> c. Imagine your breath as a stream of light or energy, entering your body with each inhalation and leaving with each exhalation.
>
> d. Visualize this stream of light or energy circulating throughout your body, nourishing and energizing every cell.
>
> e. Practice for five minutes, focusing on the visualization of your breath.

Breath Synchronization with Movement Exercise:

> a. Stand with your feet hip-width apart and arms at your sides.

b. Inhale deeply, raising your arms overhead.

c. Exhale, bending forward at the hips, and bringing your hands to the floor or your shins.

d. Inhale, lifting your chest halfway up, creating a flat back.

e. Exhale, folding forward again.

f. Inhale, raising your arms overhead, and returning to the starting position.

g. Practice for five minutes, focusing on synchronizing your breath with each movement.

Using Pranayama to Connect with Your Inner Light

Think about your inner light - the unique spark that makes you, you. It's there, always, within you, waiting to be connected with on a whole new level. Guess what? Pranayama can help you do just that.

A Journey to Improved Health and Vitality

When I first started weaving movement techniques into the tapestry of my daily routine, my driving force was a longing to boost my physical health. My brother, a fitness enthusiast, recommended that I try incorporating yoga and tai chi into my mornings. With a bit of reluctance, I agreed, thinking it was yet another passing trend in the fitness world.

But as the calendar pages turned, I stumbled upon a newfound wellspring of energy and vitality. My chronic back pain diminished, and I felt more flexible and agile than I had in years. What began as an experiment to appease my brother transformed into a lifelong passion for the power of movement and its ability to heal the body and mind.

Ready to connect with your inner light? Let's dive into this guided meditation practice using Ujjayi Pranayama.

Your Personal Guide: Visualizing Your Inner Light with Ujjayi Pranayama

Find a comfortable seated position. You may choose to sit cross-legged on the floor or on a cushion, or in a chair with your feet flat on the ground.

Close your eyes and take a few deep breaths to settle into the present moment.

Begin to practice Ujjayi breathing by inhaling and exhaling through your nose while constricting the back of your throat. This will create a soft, hissing sound in the back of your throat.

Take a few rounds of Ujjayi breaths, focusing on the sound and sensation of the breath moving in and out of your body.

Visualize a radiant light at your heart center, representing your inner light. Imagine this light as warm and bright, filling your entire chest cavity. As you focus on this light, feel the warmth enveloping your body, transporting you to a serene, peaceful place where you can connect with your true self.

With each inhalation, imagine this light expanding and brightening, filling your entire body. Allow the light to spread outwards from your heart center, bathing your entire body in a warm, golden glow.

With each exhalation, imagine any negativity, stress, or tension leaving your body. Imagine the light carrying away any negative emotions or sensations, leaving you feeling calm and peaceful.

Continue practicing Ujjayi breathing while focusing on your visualization of the inner light. Try to maintain your focus on the visualization and your breath for at least five minutes.

When you are ready to end the practice, take a few deep breaths and bring your attention back to your physical surroundings. Open your eyes and take a moment to notice how you feel after the practice.

A Shared Experience of Transformation

One of the most heart-warming chapters in my breathwork and movement journey has been seeing the transformative power it has had on other people's lives. I recall hosting a small workshop for a group of people who were facing various personal challenges. Among them was a woman named Linda, who had been grappling with intense anxiety and depression for years.

As we practiced deep belly breathing and gentle movements, I noticed a visible shift in Linda's demeanor. By the end of the session, she shared with the group how the techniques had helped her feel more present and connected to her body for the first time in years. Her story is just one of many that have inspired me to continue sharing these transformative techniques with others, and it's a testament to the power of breath and movement in creating lasting change.

Linda's experience demonstrates the potential of breathwork and movement techniques, like Ujjayi breathing and visualization of inner light, to create lasting change and bring a sense of inner calm, clarity, and focus into our daily lives.

I am grateful for the opportunity to practice yoga and pranayama. The techniques have changed my life, helping me find inner peace and balance in my hectic daily routine. I now have a deeper connection to my body, mind, and spirit." - Emma, yoga and pranayama practitioner

Leveraging Movement to Let Go of Tension

Movement, my friends, is a potent ally in our yoga practice. It helps release tension and stress while improving flexibility and strength. What would it mean for you to be able to release tension in your body and mind through simple, intentional movements? Imagine the possibilities for greater relaxation and ease in your life.

By engaging in specific yoga poses and sequences, you can calm your mind and bring yourself into the present moment. Here are some yoga poses and sequences that can help you release tension:

Cat-Cow Sequence:

a. Begin on your hands and knees, with your hands directly under your shoulders and your knees under your hips.

b. Inhale, arching your back and lifting your chest and tailbone toward the sky (Cow Pose).

c. Exhale, rounding your back, tucking your tailbone under, and bringing your chin toward your chest (Cat Pose).

d. Continue this sequence for five to ten breaths, focusing on the rhythm of your breath and the movement of your spine.

Forward Fold Sequence:

a. Stand with your feet hip-width apart, arms at your sides.

b. Inhale, raising your arms overhead.

c. Exhale, bending forward at the hips, bringing your hands to the floor or your shins.

d. Inhale, lifting your chest halfway up, creating a flat back.

e. Exhale, folding forward again.

f. Inhale, raising your arms overhead, and returning to the starting position.

g. Practice for five minutes, focusing on the breath and the release of tension in your hamstrings and lower back.

Sun Salutations:

a. Stand with your feet together, arms at your sides.

b. Inhale, raising your arms overhead.

c. Exhale, folding forward at the hips, bringing your hands to the floor or your shins.

d. Inhale, stepping your right foot back into a lunge, keeping your left knee bent and your right leg straight.

e. Exhale, stepping your left foot back into a plank position.

f. On your next inhale, lower your body into Chaturanga Dandasana (Four-Limbed Staff Pose), keeping your elbows close to your body.

g. On the following exhale, press into your hands and lift your hips, transitioning into Downward-Facing Dog.

h. Inhale, stepping your right foot forward into a lunge, keeping your left leg straight and your right knee bent.

i. Exhale, stepping your left foot forward, coming into a forward fold.

j. Inhale, raising your arms overhead, and returning to the starting position.

k. Repeat on the other side.

l. Practice for five minutes, focusing on the breath and the fluidity of the movements.

Unraveling the Deep-Seated Connection Between Mind and Body

Getting to know and bolstering the bond between your mind and body is a key player in personal growth and holistic well-being. How could these practices transform your daily life?

Are you ready to explore the power of your mind-body connection to create positive change? By becoming more aware of this connection, you can harness its power to transform your life. Here are some self-assessment techniques to help you evaluate and strengthen your mind-body connection:

Body Scan Meditation:

a. Find a comfortable seated or lying position.

b. Close your eyes and take a few deep breaths to center yourself.

c. Begin scanning your body, starting at your toes and working your way up to the crown of your head.

d. Pay attention to any sensations, tension, or discomfort in each body part.

e. Practice for 10-15 minutes, focusing on your breath and the sensations in your body.

Journaling Exercise:

a. Set aside 10-15 minutes each day for journaling.

b. Write about your thoughts, feelings, and experiences during your yoga and pranayama practice.

c. Reflect on any patterns or insights you discover regarding your mind-body connection.

d. Use this information to make adjustments in your practice and daily life.

Mindful Movement Practice:

a. Choose a simple physical activity (such as walking, stretching, or doing household chores) to practice mindfulness.

b. As you engage in the activity, focus on the sensations in your body and the movement itself.

c. Notice any thoughts or emotions that arise and observe them without judgment.

d. Continue this practice for 10-15 minutes, cultivating a deeper awareness of your mind-body connection.

Incorporating interactive elements such as exercises, self-assessments, and guided meditations into your yoga and pranayama practice can enrich your experience and deepen your understanding of the techniques.

By cultivating breath awareness and control, connecting with your inner light, releasing tension through movement, and strengthening your mind-body connection, you will empower yourself to achieve balance, mindfulness, and fulfillment in your daily life.

All the techniques discussed in this chapter, from connecting with your inner light to releasing tension through movement, contribute to a holistic approach to well-being and personal growth. By practicing these techniques consistently, you'll cultivate a stronger connection between your body and mind, enabling you to tap into your inner resources for lasting transformation.

Embrace the transformative power of breath and movement. By integrating these practices into your daily life, you'll foster mental clarity, emotional balance, and physical strength. The journey to personal growth and self-discovery begins with a single step. Don't wait for tomorrow; take that step now. Commit to the techniques that resonate with you and cultivate a lifestyle of balance, mindfulness, and fulfillment. Remember, the light within you is waiting to shine. Let it illuminate your path to a more mindful, balanced, and fulfilled life.

5

Embracing Fearlessness: Overcoming Fear and Judgment in Life

The Impact of Fear and Judgment on Our Lives: Discovering the Power of Mindfulness

Imagine yourself in the midst of everyday chaos, bombarded by honking cars, chattering crowds, and the relentless hustle of life. As if emerging from the depths of a stormy sea, a practice like a beacon of light guides you towards tranquility and balance. Mindfulness, a simple yet profound practice, became my compass, steering me through turbulent waters and into the calm harbor of self-awareness.

At first, I was skeptical. How could something as seemingly simple as mindfulness have such a significant impact on my daily life? Through daily practice, I began to see the effects of mindfulness ripple throughout my life. I found that I was more patient, more understanding, and more compassionate, both towards myself and others. My relationships deepened, my work became more fulfilling, and my overall sense of well-being soared to new heights. By fostering a deep sense of self-awareness and presence, mindfulness can help us confront and overcome the fears and judgments that often hold us back in life.

Incorporating Mindfulness Practices into Daily Life (section combined with the previous passage)

So, how can you begin to incorporate mindfulness practices into your daily life? Let me share some techniques that have worked wonders for me and countless others:

- Start with meditation
- Practice yoga
- Mindful eating
- Engage in mindful activities
- Practice gratitude

As you embark on your own journey towards mindfulness, remember that it is a lifelong practice. There will be days when it feels challenging, and there will be days when it feels effortless. But with each mindful breath and every present moment, you are nurturing a deep connection to yourself and the world around you, transforming your daily life into a rich tapestry of experience and growth.

The Power of Mindfulness in Overcoming Fear and Judgment

In this chapter, we will explore how mindfulness practices, particularly yoga, can serve as powerful tools to help us overcome the limiting effects of fear and judgment, guiding us towards a more fulfilling, authentic life. I recall a time when my own fear of failure held me back from pursuing my passion for writing. It wasn't until I began practicing mindfulness that I was able to face and overcome this fear, ultimately leading me to a more authentic and fulfilling path.

My own journey towards embracing mindfulness began with a struggle. For years, I found myself trapped in a cycle of fear and self-judgment, constantly questioning my worth and abilities. That's when I discovered yoga, a practice that would ultimately transform my life.

As I deepened my connection to the practice, I found solace and strength on my yoga mat. With each breath and movement, I learned to quiet the whispers of self-doubt and face my fears. Over time, yoga became a sanctuary for self-discovery and growth, empowering me to break the chains that once held me captive.

To dive deeper into the transformative power of mindfulness practices, let us examine case studies of individuals who have successfully overcome fear and judgment:

A middle-aged man, once consumed by a fear of public speaking, turned to yoga and meditation to build confidence and self-compassion. Over time, he learned to embrace vulnerability, eventually becoming a renowned motivational speaker.

A single mother, struggling with feelings of inadequacy and the fear of judgment from others, found solace and strength through yoga. As her practice deepened, she discovered the resilience within herself, creating a more balanced and fulfilling life for her

Building a Fearless and Non-judgmental Mindset

In a small village, a wise monk named Master Tenzin cultivated a fearless and non-judgmental mindset through years of mindfulness practice. Let's explore the impact of mindfulness on daily life and learn how to build our own fearless and non-judgmental mindset.

The sun had barely risen when Master Tenzin began his daily routine. He would start with a gentle walk through the village, observing the beauty and simplicity of the world around him. With each step, he practiced mindfulness, staying fully present in the moment, and acknowledging his thoughts and emotions without judgment. This simple act of walking meditation helped him maintain a clear and focused mind throughout the day.

Mindful breathing: One of the easiest ways to practice mindfulness is by focusing on your breath. Close your eyes, take a deep breath in through your nose, and slowly exhale through your mouth. As you breathe, notice the sensations in your body and the thoughts that arise in your mind. Acknowledge them without judgment and gently bring your focus back to your breath.

Body scan meditation: Lie down in a comfortable position and bring your attention to your toes. Gradually move your focus up through your legs, torso, arms, and head, noticing any sensations or tension you might be experiencing. As you become aware of these feelings, imagine them melting away, leaving your body relaxed and at ease.

Loving-kindness meditation: In this practice, you'll cultivate feelings of love and compassion for yourself and others. Start by silently repeating phrases such as "May I be happy, may I be healthy, may I be safe, may I live with ease," and gradually expand your focus to include friends, family, and even those with whom you may have difficulties.

Now, let me share a personal experience that illustrates the power of cultivating a fearless and non-judgmental mindset. A few years ago, I found myself in a challenging work situation. My boss was demanding and critical, and my colleagues were often unsupportive. I felt overwhelmed and defeated. Then, I began practicing mindfulness, focusing on my breath and incorporating loving-kindness meditation into my daily routine. Slowly but surely, my mindset began to shift.

Instead of dwelling on my perceived failures, I learned to accept my emotions and thoughts without judgment. I became more resilient in the face of criticism and embraced challenges with courage and curiosity. My relationships with my colleagues improved, and my work environment became more harmonious. I had discovered the transformative power of a fearless and non-judgmental mindset, and it changed my life for the better.

In the same way that Master Tenzin's daily mindfulness practice enabled him to maintain equanimity and grace, we too can reap the benefits of a fearless and non-judgmental mindset. By incorporating mindfulness practices into our daily lives, we can foster greater resilience, compassion, and joy in the face of life's challenges. So, take a deep breath, embrace the present moment, and let's embark on this journey together.

Now that we've discussed the impact of mindfulness on overcoming fear and judgment, let's dive into some specific techniques and tips to help you on your journey.

Techniques to Foster Fearlessness

Cultivating a fearless mindset enables you to face challenges with courage and resilience. Let's explore techniques and practices to help you develop fearlessness.

Technique 1: Embrace the Power of Visualization

Visualization is a powerful tool for fostering fearlessness. By mentally rehearsing a challenging situation, you can train your brain to respond with courage and confidence. Here's how:

In a quiet space, visualize yourself facing a fear-inducing situation and responding with courage and confidence.

Picture yourself facing a situation that evokes fear, such as public speaking or confronting a difficult conversation.

Visualize yourself responding with courage, grace, and confidence.

Feel the fear dissipating as you take control of the situation.

Technique 2: Develop a Growth Mindset

A growth mindset is the belief that abilities and intelligence can be developed through dedication and hard work. By adopting this mindset, you can view challenges as opportunities for growth, fostering fearlessness in the face of adversity.

Reflect on past experiences where you overcame fear or faced challenges.

Identify the skills and strategies you used to succeed in those situations.

Remind yourself that every challenge is an opportunity to learn and grow.

Technique 3: Practice Mindful Yoga

Yoga is an ancient practice that unites the mind, body, and spirit, promoting fearlessness by cultivating inner strength and resilience. Incorporate the following yoga poses into your daily routine to foster fearlessness:

Warrior Pose (Virabhadrasana): This powerful standing pose builds strength, balance, and focus.

Tree Pose (Vrikshasana): This balancing pose fosters stability and mental clarity.

Lion's Breath (Simhasana): This seated pose releases tension and fear through a powerful exhale.

By incorporating these techniques into your daily life, you can cultivate a fearless mindset that empowers you to face challenges head-on. Remember, fear is a natural response to the unknown, but with practice and dedication, you can transform it into an unstoppable force for growth and resilience. So take a deep breath, embrace the present moment, and step boldly into the unknown.

As we continue our exploration, let's focus on practical tips and advice for incorporating non-judgmental thinking into your daily routines and interactions.

Embracing Non-judgment in Daily Life

Cultivating Mindful Awareness through Active Listening

Non-judgmental thinking is a crucial aspect of mindfulness that can have a profound impact on our daily lives. Let's explore practical tips for incorporating non-judgmental thinking into your daily routines and interactions.

In this section, we will explore practical tips and advice for incorporating non-judgmental thinking into your daily routines and interactions. By embracing a non-judgmental mindset, you can cultivate greater empathy, compassion, and understanding, fostering deeper connections with yourself and others.

Tip 1: Cultivate Mindful Awareness through Active Listening: One of the most effective ways to cultivate non-judgment in daily life is by practicing active listening while also developing mindful awareness. This means fully engaging with the speaker, giving them your undivided attention, and withholding judgment as they share their thoughts and feelings. Set aside distractions such as phones or other devices. Maintain eye contact and open body language. Reflect back what you heard and ask open-ended questions to encourage further discussion. Meanwhile, practice mindfulness by focusing on your breath, bodily sensations, or thoughts. Acknowledge any judgmental thoughts without engaging with them or assigning value. Gently redirect your attention to the present moment, maintaining an attitude of curiosity and openness.

Challenging Your Assumptions

Tip 2: Challenge Your Assumptions

Often, judgment arises from deeply ingrained beliefs or assumptions about ourselves, others, and the world around us. By actively challenging these beliefs, we can create space for non-judgmental thinking to take root.

Identify any recurring judgmental thoughts or patterns in your life.

Examine the underlying beliefs or assumptions that give rise to these judgments.

Consider alternative perspectives, and be open to the possibility of changing your beliefs or assumptions.

Practicing Empathy and Compassion

Tip 3: Practice Empathy and Compassion

Embracing non-judgment in daily life means cultivating empathy and compassion, both for ourselves and others. By seeking to understand the experiences and perspectives of others, we can foster a greater sense of connection and acceptance.

Put yourself in another person's shoes, imagining their feelings, thoughts, and experiences.

Acknowledge that everyone has their unique journey, and that their perspective is valid, even if it differs from your own.

Extend compassion and understanding to yourself, recognizing that your own thoughts and feelings are worthy of acceptance, even if they are not in alignment with your ideals.

By incorporating these tips and practices into your daily life, you can foster a non-judgmental mindset that allows you to navigate the complexities of human interaction with grace, compassion, and understanding. Remember, the journey toward non-judgment is an ongoing process, requiring patience and persistence. But with each mindful step, you will find yourself more connected to the present moment, more open to the richness of human experience, and more able to embrace the world with an open heart.

Unleashing Your Inner Strength

Yoga is an ancient practice that unites the mind, body, and spirit, serving as a powerful catalyst for personal transformation. It offers a unique pathway to inner strength, allowing us to cultivate resilience, focus, and equanimity amidst the challenges of daily life. By embracing the wisdom and discipline of yoga, we can embark on a journey of self-discovery, awakening the inherent power that lies within.

The beauty of yoga lies in its ability to adapt to the needs of each individual, offering a diverse array of practices that cater to a wide range of abilities and preferences. From the dynamic flow of Vinyasa to the meditative stillness of Yin, there is a style of yoga to suit every seeker on the path to inner strength.

As you delve into your yoga practice, you may find yourself exploring various techniques, each offering its own unique benefits. Some of these techniques may include:

Physical Asanas: The practice of physical postures, or asanas, helps to build strength, flexibility, and balance, forging a strong connection between the body and mind. As you challenge yourself to hold poses and move through sequences, you cultivate a sense of resilience and determination that carries over into other aspects of your life.

Breathwork: By focusing on the breath, we can cultivate a sense of inner calm and presence, even in the face of adversity. Practices such as pranayama, or breath control, help to regulate the flow of energy within the body, promoting clarity, focus, and emotional stability.

Meditation: The practice of meditation encourages mindfulness and self-awareness, allowing us to tap into our inner reservoir of strength and wisdom. By cultivating a focused and non-judgmental awareness of our thoughts and emotions, we can learn to navigate life's challenges with grace and equanimity.

The path to inner strength is not linear, but with each mindful breath, deliberate movement, and moment of stillness, you nurture resilience and courage within.

Yoga for Emotional Release and Resilience

In the tapestry of life, we often encounter a myriad of emotions, weaving together a rich and complex narrative that shapes our experiences. At times, we may find ourselves grappling with challenging emotions, weighed down by the burden of stress, anxiety, or grief. Yet, through the practice of yoga, we can learn to release these emotions and cultivate resilience, empowering us to navigate life's challenges with grace and equanimity.

Yoga for emotional release and resilience focuses on the connection between the mind, body, and spirit, using a combination of physical postures, breathwork, and meditation to access and release stored emotions. By embracing this holistic approach, we can cultivate a greater sense of balance and harmony, fostering emotional resilience in the face of adversity.

In this section, we will explore how yoga can help us release challenging emotions and build resilience through specific poses, breathwork, and awareness. By incorporating these practices into your yoga routine, you can create a powerful means for emotional healing and growth.

In this section, we will explore several key yoga poses that can help release emotions and build resilience. These poses, combined with mindful breathing and awareness, can create a powerful practice for emotional healing and growth.

1. **Child's Pose (Balasana):** This gentle, restorative pose allows you to turn inward and connect with your innermost feelings. By surrendering to the earth, you create a safe space for emotional release and introspection.
2. **Pigeon Pose (Eka Pada Rajakapotasana):** This deep hip opener can help release stored emotions, particularly those associated with stress, anxiety, and past traumas. By allowing the hips to open and soften, we create an opportunity for emotional healing and release.
3. **Supported Bridge Pose (Setu Bandha Sarvangasana):** This gentle backbend helps to alleviate stress and anxiety while promoting relaxation. Unlike the standard Bridge Pose, which focuses on strengthening the back muscles and opening the chest, the supported variation places a prop such as a yoga block or bolster underneath the sacrum, allowing for a more restorative experience and encouraging the release of tension and emotional blockages.

As you explore these poses and delve deeper into your yoga practice, you may find that the process of emotional release and resilience unfolds organically, like the unfurling of a delicate flower. Each breath, movement, and moment of stillness offers an opportunity for healing and growth, allowing you to reclaim your power and embrace the full spectrum of human experience.

Remember, the journey toward emotional release and resilience is a deeply personal and unique path, shaped by your own experiences and intentions. Be gentle with yourself as you navigate this transformative process, knowing that with each step, you are fostering a greater sense of inner strength and resilience that will serve as a beacon of light amidst the ever-changing landscape of life.

Guided Meditation: Conquering Fear and Judgment

As we delve deeper into the world of mindfulness and its impact on daily life, it's important to remember that fear and judgment are natural emotions that everyone encounters. However, through guided meditation, we can learn to conquer these feelings, allowing ourselves to live with greater freedom and authenticity. In this section, we'll explore a step-by-step guided meditation designed to help you address fears and judgments, empowering you to cultivate a fearless and non-judgmental mindset.

Before we begin, find a comfortable and quiet space where you can sit or lie down without distractions. Allow yourself to fully immerse in the meditation, knowing that this is your time for self-care and introspection.

Step 1: Settle into your meditation posture

Begin by sitting or lying down in a comfortable position, allowing your spine to maintain its natural alignment. Close your eyes gently and take a few deep, cleansing breaths. As you exhale, imagine any tension or stress melting away from your body.

Step 2: Grounding and centering

As you continue to breathe, bring your attention to the sensation of your body making contact with the surface beneath you. Feel the support of the earth, as if roots were extending from your body, grounding and centering you in this present moment.

Step 3: Mindful breathing

Begin to focus on your breath, noticing the natural rhythm of your inhales and exhales. Pay attention to the sensation of the air entering and leaving your nostrils or the rise and fall of your chest. If your mind begins to wander, gently guide it back to the breath, without judgment.

Step 4: Visualization of a safe space

Imagine a serene and peaceful place that brings you a sense of comfort and safety. This could be a tranquil beach, a lush forest, or a cozy room filled with warm light. Allow yourself to be fully immersed in this safe space, feeling protected and at ease.

Step 5: Facing your fears

As you continue to breathe deeply and effortlessly, envision your fears and judgments appearing in front of you, taking the form of clouds or balloons. Observe them without attachment or judgment, acknowledging their presence.

Step 6: Letting go

With each exhale, imagine your fears and judgments dissipating or floating away, leaving you with a sense of peace and lightness. Continue this process until you feel a deep sense of release and freedom from these emotions.

Step 7: Cultivating compassion and understanding

Now, envision a warm, healing light enveloping you, filling you with love, compassion, and understanding. Allow this light to expand within you, connecting you with your inner strength and resilience, empowering you to face your fears and judgments with courage and acceptance.

Step 8: Returning to the present moment

Gradually bring your awareness back to your breath and the sensation of your body making contact with the surface beneath you. As you feel ready, gently open your eyes and take a moment to acknowledge the journey you've just experienced.

Remember that meditation is a personal and unique process, and it's perfectly normal to encounter challenges or distractions along the way. Be gentle with yourself and embrace the practice with an open heart, knowing that each meditation session is an opportunity for growth and self-discovery. By regularly engaging in this guided meditation, you'll cultivate a fearless and non-judgmental mindset, empowering you to navigate the complexities of daily life with grace and equanimity.

Tools and Techniques for Letting Go of Limiting Beliefs

Recognize your limiting beliefs:

The initial step in overcoming limiting beliefs is to identify them. Contemplate the areas of your life where you feel restricted or stagnant. What beliefs could be causing these feelings? Write them down to gain clarity and heighten your self-awareness.

To better understand and address your limiting beliefs, consider incorporating the following tools and techniques into your daily routine:

- Challenge and reframe your thoughts
- Positive affirmations
- Harness the power of visualization
- Emotional Freedom Technique (EFT)
- Practice mindfulness and self-compassion

By actively exploring and applying these techniques, you can work towards releasing limiting beliefs and opening yourself up to a life filled with greater freedom, authenticity, and happiness.

Challenge and reframe your thoughts:

Cognitive restructuring is a valuable technique that involves identifying and challenging negative or irrational thoughts. When a limiting belief arises, question whether it's based on fact or assumption. Then, reframe the thought in a more optimistic and realistic light.

Positive affirmations:

Using affirmations—positive statements that counteract negative self-talk and reinforce healthier beliefs—can have a transformative impact on your mindset. Develop affirmations that target your limiting beliefs and recite them daily to reshape your thought patterns.

Harness the power of visualization:

Visualization is a potent tool for overcoming limiting beliefs. Imagine yourself liberated from the beliefs constraining you and envision the life you would lead without these limitations. Regular practice will reinforce the idea that you can conquer your limiting beliefs and accomplish your goals.

Emotional Freedom Technique (EFT):

EFT, or "tapping," is a technique that blends acupressure and psychology to release emotional blockages. Tapping on specific energy points while concentrating on a limiting belief allows your body and mind to release the associated emotional charge, making it easier to let go of the belief.

Practice mindfulness and self-compassion:

Develop a mindfulness practice that encourages self-compassion and non-judgment. By fostering awareness of your thoughts and emotions, you can learn to recognize limiting beliefs without becoming entangled in them. Embrace self-compassion as you work through your beliefs, understanding that change requires time and effort.

As you explore and apply these tools and techniques, remember that releasing limiting beliefs is an ongoing process that necessitates patience, persistence, and self-compassion. By actively engaging in this journey, you'll open yourself up to a life filled with greater freedom, authenticity, and happiness.

Now that we have established the importance of mindfulness and self-compassion, let's delve deeper into how embarking on a journey towards a fearless and non-judgmental mindset can be life-changing. Developing a deeper understanding of your fears and judgments and learning to let go of them can pave the way for personal growth and a more fulfilling life. In this section, we'll explore various exercises, techniques, and practices designed to help you overcome your fears and judgments, ultimately leading you to a more empowered and authentic way of living.

Interactive Exercise: Fear and Judgment Reflection

In our journey towards a fearless and non-judgmental mindset, it's important to recognize and let go of limiting beliefs that hold us back. These beliefs may stem from past experiences, societal expectations, or self-doubt, but they can be transformed through mindfulness practices and intentional self-reflection. Here are some tools and techniques to help you let go of limiting beliefs and embrace your true potential:

Journaling: Writing down your thoughts, feelings, and beliefs can help you gain clarity and identify patterns in your thinking. Take some time each day to write about your fears, judgments, and limiting beliefs, and explore how they might be holding you back. Reflect on possible steps to overcome these beliefs and move forward.

Affirmations: Positive statements can help rewire your thought patterns and replace limiting beliefs with empowering ones. Write down a list of positive affirmations that resonate with you, such as "I am capable," "I am worthy," or "I am strong." Repeat these affirmations daily, either aloud or silently, to reinforce their power.

Mindfulness meditation: Practicing mindfulness meditation can help you become more aware of your thoughts and beliefs, allowing you to recognize and let go of those that no longer serve you. Set aside time each day to sit in a quiet space, focus on your breath, and observe your thoughts without judgment.

Deepening the Reflection on Fears and Judgments

To help you identify and analyze your own fears and judgments, try this reflection exercise:

Find a quiet, comfortable space where you can sit or lie down undisturbed for at least 15 minutes.

Close your eyes and take several deep breaths, inhaling through your nose and exhaling through your mouth. Allow your body and mind to relax as you settle into the present moment.

As you continue to breathe deeply, begin to reflect on your fears and judgments. What are the sources of these fears? How do they manifest in your daily life? Are there specific situations or people that trigger them?

Now, consider the impact of these fears and judgments on your life. How do they limit you? How might your life be different if you could let go of them?

Finally, imagine yourself releasing these fears and judgments, one by one. Visualize them floating away like balloons or dissolving into the air. Feel the weight lifting from your shoulders and your heart opening up to new possibilities.

When you're ready, take a few more deep breaths and slowly open your eyes. Record your insights and reflections in a journal, noting any patterns or themes that emerge.

Remember, this exercise is meant to be an honest and open exploration of your inner world. The more you practice, the better equipped you'll be to identify and let go of limiting beliefs and embrace a fearless, non-judgmental mindset.

Self-Assessment: Identifying Personal Fears and Judgments

In this section of our journey through mindfulness and its impact on daily life, we're going to delve into the realm of personal fears and judgments. These internal barriers can impede our growth and well-being, making it essential to recognize and address them. Here, we'll present a self-assessment that will assist you in identifying your fears and judgments, as well as understanding how they affect your life. With this newfound self-awareness, you'll be better prepared to confront these challenges and progress towards a more fulfilling life.

Self-Assessment: Uncovering Personal Fears and Judgments

- **Engage in introspection:** Set aside some time to reflect on your life and the various experiences you've encountered. Focus on situations involving fear or judgment towards yourself, others, or circumstances.
- **Examine your judgments:** Next, consider any judgments you've made about yourself, others, or situations. These might relate to appearance, behavior, beliefs, or anything else that comes to mind. Note these judgments, striving for specificity.
- **Evaluate the consequences:** Reflect on how the fears and judgments you've documented have influenced your thoughts, emotions, and actions. For instance, have your fears prevented you from chasing your dreams? Have your judgments generated discord or strife in your relationships?
- **Organize your fears and judgments:** To gain deeper insight into the nature of your fears and judgments, arrange them into categories. You may have fears related to social interactions, self-esteem, or failure, for example. Likewise, your judgments could be sorted by themes like appearance, intelligence, or values.
- **Set your priorities:** Review your categorized list and decide which fears and judgments you'd like to tackle first. Prioritizing will help you concentrate your efforts and maximize your personal growth.

Upon completing this self-assessment, you'll possess a better understanding of your personal fears and judgments and the ways they affect your life. With this information at hand, you can begin the process of releasing these limiting beliefs and adopting a more mindful, empathetic, and satisfying way of living.

As you continue to practice mindfulness and engage in self-exploration, you'll discover that your fears and judgments lose their power, enabling you to live more genuinely and experience the profound advantages of mindfulness in your daily life.

Embracing the Power of Non-Attachment

In our ongoing journey toward self-discovery and personal growth, it is vital to delve into the concept of non-attachment. Non-attachment, an empowering mindfulness practice, releases fears, judgments, and limiting beliefs, leading to increased inner peace, satisfaction, and liberation.

Understanding Non-Attachment

Non-attachment involves letting go of our emotional and mental hold on people, situations, and results. It signifies cultivating an open, adaptable, and accepting mindset to tackle life's challenges with composure and resilience, not indifference or lack of concern. Practicing non-attachment moves beyond fears and judgments, recognizing them as temporary, unhelpful mental constructs.

A Step-by-Step Guide: Incorporating Non-Attachment into Daily Life

- **Embrace impermanence:** Accept that everything in life is transient and prone to change. Welcome this reality and remind yourself that clinging to any particular outcome or situation is unproductive.
- **Cultivate self-compassion:** Treat yourself with kindness as you navigate the process of non-attachment. Remember that releasing attachment is a skill that requires time and practice to develop.
- **Let go of control:** Acknowledge that you can't control everything in life. Relinquish the need to control outcomes and trust that things will ultimately unfold as they should.

- **Practical Guidance:** Integrating Non-Attachment into Everyday Habits and Decision-Making
- **Establish realistic expectations:** When setting objectives or making plans, be pragmatic about what you can accomplish and avoid becoming excessively attached to specific outcomes.
- **Accept uncertainty:** Learn to be at ease with uncertainty and embrace the unknown. This mindset will help you manage change and make decisions without being constrained by attachment to particular outcomes.
- **Practice gratitude:** Concentrate on the present moment and express gratitude for what you have, rather than focusing on what you lack or desire to change.
- **Nurture healthy relationships:** Apply non-attachment in your relationships by allowing others the space and freedom to be themselves, without attempting to control or influence their actions or emotions.
- **Assess your progress:** Regularly evaluate your development in practicing non-attachment and recognize your growth while also identifying areas where you can continue to evolve.

Embrace this transformative practice, and observe as it unveils new avenues for personal growth, self-discovery, and a more enriching existence.

Meditation Techniques and Positive Affirmations for a Fearless and Non-judgmental Mind

Meditation is a powerful practice that can help cultivate a fearless and non-judgmental mindset. Some effective meditation techniques include mindfulness meditation, loving-kindness meditation, and body scan meditation. Mindfulness meditation teaches us to be present and aware of our thoughts and emotions without judgment, while loving-kindness meditation focuses on developing compassion and love for ourselves and others. Body scan meditation, on the other hand, encourages self-awareness and relaxation by guiding us through a mental scan of our body.

Positive affirmations can also play a vital role in overcoming fear and judgment. Repeating empowering statements can help rewire our thought patterns and reinforce fearlessness and non-judgmental thinking. Some examples of positive affirmations include:

- "I am worthy of love and respect."
- "I release fear and embrace courage."
- "I am open to new experiences and growth."

Building a Supportive Environment

Surrounding ourselves with supportive individuals and environments is essential for fostering fearlessness and non-judgment. Engage with people who encourage your personal growth, and distance yourself from those who perpetuate fear and judgment. One example of this is Jane, who found that joining a yoga community helped her overcome her fear of judgment and allowed her to feel accepted and supported.

Self-Compassion and Daily Practices for a Fearless and Non-judgmental Life

Self-compassion is crucial for overcoming fear and judgment. Treat yourself with kindness and understanding, and remember that it is okay to make mistakes.

- Acknowledging your emotions without judgment
- Practicing self-forgiveness
- Reminding yourself of your strengths and accomplishments

Incorporating daily practices and habits that support a fearless and non-judgmental mindset can have a significant impact on your overall well-being. Some of these practices include:

- Regular meditation and mindfulness exercises
- Journaling to reflect on your thoughts and emotions
- Engaging in physical activities that promote relaxation and self-awareness, such as yoga

Embracing a Life Free of Fear and Judgment

Embracing a life free of fear and judgment is a transformative journey that involves meditation, positive affirmations, supportive environments, self-compassion, and daily practices. Consider the story of John, who overcame his fear of public speaking through yoga and mindfulness, ultimately leading him to become a confident and inspiring speaker. By incorporating these strategies into your life, you too can cultivate a fearless and non-judgmental mindset that allows you to thrive and grow.

In this chapter, we have explored various tools, techniques, and practices designed to help you overcome fears and judgments. By implementing these strategies consistently, you can experience significant personal growth and lead a more fulfilling life. Remember that progress is a journey, and with patience, persistence, and self-compassion, you'll continue to evolve and break free from the chains of fear and judgment.

6

Embracing Your Inner Shine: Discovering Your Unique Gifts and Talents. Understanding the Importance of Your Inner Shine

Life's journey often unveils our unique 'Inner Shine', the essence of who we are. It's the manifestation of our gifts, talents, and potential, illuminating our path and guiding us towards our purpose.

Unlocking this inner shine, akin to unearthing a hidden treasure within us, leads to transformation, growth, and fulfillment. It's a treasure often overlooked or suppressed by fear, judgment, or self-doubt.

John, introduced in the previous chapter, is a prime example of discovering one's inner shine. Initially, his public speaking talent was veiled by fear, but yoga and mindfulness helped him confront this fear, dissolve self-doubt, and reveal his inner shine.

Recognizing and harnessing our inner shine requires self-awareness and acceptance, acknowledging our talents and strengths as guides in our pursuits, while viewing our weaknesses not as limitations, but growth and learning opportunities.

Your inner shine, the essence of who you are, acts as a beacon, expressing your individuality and revealing your unique gifts and talents.

Appreciating and nurturing our inner shine helps cultivate a life of authenticity, purpose, and fulfillment, a profound journey requiring patience, persistence, and self-compassion.

As we embrace our inner shine, we not only grow as individuals but also contribute our unique light to the world, making it a brighter place. So, let your inner shine illuminate your path, and see where it leads you. Your journey is just beginning.

Personal Stories and Anecdotes

Every person's unique story, woven from experiences, strengths, and passions, is the fingerprint of their Inner Shine, the radiant essence of who they are. Let's delve into a couple of stories that illustrate the transformative power of embracing our unique gifts and talents.

Consider Lisa, a highly skilled violinist. From a young age, she showed an uncanny ability to express emotions through music. However, Lisa spent most of her life hiding this talent, believing it was insignificant. She pursued a conventional career path, becoming an accountant. It was a secure job, yet it left her feeling unfulfilled and disconnected from herself.

One day, Lisa reluctantly agreed to perform at a friend's wedding. As she played, the room fell silent. The audience was captivated by her performance, moved by the emotional depth and beauty of the music. The experience was transformative for Lisa. She realized that her unique talent for music wasn't insignificant; it was her Inner Shine, a powerful expression of her individuality. Lisa decided to honor her gift, eventually transitioning from her accounting career to becoming a professional violinist. Today, she not only finds fulfillment in her work but also brings joy to others through her music. Her

Inner Shine has grown brighter, enhancing her life and positively influencing those around her.

Can you relate to Lisa's experience? Have you ever dismissed a talent of yours as insignificant? Consider how acknowledging and nurturing that talent could enhance your life and those around you.

Now, let's consider Alex. Alex was always the person his friends turned to when they needed advice or a listening ear. He had a knack for understanding people's emotions and situations. Yet, Alex never saw this as a unique talent. Instead, he saw it as a simple act of friendship.

Professionally, Alex was an engineer, a role seldom requiring his empathetic nature. Over time, a growing sense of dissatisfaction set in. He yearned for a role that would allow him to connect with people on a deeper level. Encouraged by a friend, he began volunteering at a local community center, offering support to individuals facing difficult situations. The experience was eye-opening for Alex. He found immense satisfaction in helping others navigate their challenges. It was a eureka moment for him: Alex discovered his unique gift for empathy was his Inner Shine.

Inspired, Alex pursued a degree in counseling, eventually transitioning from engineering to a career as a therapist. Today, Alex's Inner Shine is brighter than ever. He has found fulfillment in his work and made a significant impact on the lives of many.

Do you see yourself in Alex's story? Are there talents or strengths you've overlooked because they felt too commonplace or 'simple'? Imagine the potential impact if you fully embraced and utilized these abilities.

These stories demonstrate the enhancement of our Inner Shine and subsequent personal growth and fulfillment when we embrace our unique gifts and talents. But remember, discovering and nurturing your Inner Shine is a journey. It requires self-awareness, self-acceptance, and the courage to step outside your comfort zone. Whether your Inner Shine is your ability to create art, solve complex problems, or empathize with others, it's a treasure worth discovering and embracing. By doing so, you'll not only enrich your own life but also positively impact those around you. Let your Inner Shine guide you, and embrace the unique story it tells.

The Role of Yoga in Discovering Your Unique Gifts and Talents

Yoga is a potent tool for self-discovery, illuminating our unique gifts and talents to enhance our Inner Shine. It's much more than a physical workout; it's a journey of self-exploration, an exercise in mindfulness, and a path to personal growth.

Consider Maya, a corporate executive caught up in her demanding job's hustle and bustle. She was successful, but she felt like she was merely existing, not truly living. Searching for balance, she turned to yoga.

Initially, Maya saw yoga as merely a physical exercise, a way to stretch and strengthen her body. But as she continued her practice, she found it was much more. The practice of yoga allowed Maya to slow down and tune into her body, her breath, and her mind. Through this mindful awareness, Maya began to understand herself on a deeper level.

During her meditative moments in yoga, she discovered a deep-seated passion for wellness and a talent for motivating others. These were aspects of herself that she had overlooked in the hustle and bustle of her corporate life. Yoga allowed her to connect with this passion and realize her potential to inspire others. This realization was her Inner Shine breaking through.

Maya decided to channel this newfound passion and talent, eventually transitioning from her corporate job to becoming a wellness coach. She now combines her business acumen with her passion for wellness, guiding others towards healthier, more balanced lifestyles. Maya's story is an inspiring example of how yoga can help us discover our unique gifts and talents, allowing our Inner Shine to radiate more brightly.

How does Maya's journey resonate with you? Have you experienced moments of deep self-discovery during your yoga practice? Consider how such moments could reveal your unique gifts and talents.

So, how does yoga facilitate this process of self-discovery? The practice of yoga encourages us to be present, to focus on the here and now. This heightened sense of awareness opens a window into our inner selves, enabling us to connect with our thoughts, feelings, and intuition. It's in these moments of stillness and introspection that we can often gain profound insights into our passions, strengths, and potential.

Furthermore, yoga fosters self-acceptance. It teaches us to accept our bodies, strengths, limitations, and unique qualities. This acceptance is the first step towards discovering and embracing our unique gifts and talents.

Yoga also cultivates resilience and determination. Holding a challenging pose or maintaining a steady breath, even when it's uncomfortable, teaches us to persevere, to push beyond our perceived limitations. This resilience can empower us to explore new interests, talents, and passions, allowing our Inner Shine to grow.

Lastly, yoga nurtures a sense of inner peace and harmony. As we balance our bodies in yoga, we also find balance in our minds, creating a sense of inner calm. This tranquility can create a fertile ground for our Inner Shine to flourish, guiding us towards our unique gifts and talents.

In essence, yoga is a powerful ally in the journey of self-discovery. It helps us tune into our inner selves, uncover our unique gifts and talents, and let our Inner Shine glow brightly. Whether you're a seasoned yogi or a beginner, consider how yoga can help you discover and embrace your unique gifts and talents. As Maya's story illustrates, the journey might just be transformative.

The Power of Yoga in Self-Discovery

Yoga, beyond being a pathway to physical health, is a catalyst for personal transformation and self-discovery, leading to the amplification of our Inner Shine.

Let's look at the journey of Paul. Paul was an introverted software engineer, always more comfortable with code than conversation. He discovered yoga as a way to combat work-related stress. However, as he continued practicing, he experienced more than just stress relief. Yoga became a mirror, reflecting his inner self.

During one particular yoga session, while in Savasana, the final relaxation pose, Paul experienced a profound moment of clarity. He realized that beneath his introverted exterior lay a talent for storytelling. He began to notice how he would often narrate his yoga practice, guiding himself through each pose with a story in his mind. This was an aspect of himself he'd never recognized before, his Inner Shine starting to glow.

Inspired by his discovery, Paul started writing. He channeled his storytelling into creating children's books, coding during the day and writing by night. His books, infused with his unique style, gained popularity, touching many young lives. His Inner Shine was no longer just a glow; it was a beacon.

How does yoga facilitate these revelations? Essentially, it provides a space for non-judgmental observation of our thoughts, feelings, and intuition. This conscious observation often reveals aspects of ourselves we might overlook in the chaos of everyday life.

The physical postures, or asanas, make us aware of our strengths and limitations. A challenging pose demonstrates our inner strength, whereas a difficult asana reveals areas for growth. Both of these insights can guide us to our unique gifts and talents.

The quiet introspection of yoga also nurtures self-acceptance. It encourages us to honor our individuality, a crucial step in recognizing and embracing our unique gifts and talents. This acceptance allows our Inner Shine to radiate more brightly.

Paul's experience testifies to the transformative power of yoga in self-discovery. Stepping onto the mat starts a journey of revealing our unique gifts and talents, thereby enhancing our Inner Shine. So, consider how yoga can illuminate your path to self-discovery. Your journey is waiting

Can you identify with Paul's transformative journey? Could there be a hidden talent within you waiting to be discovered? Reflect on how yoga could become a mirror for you to see your own Inner Shine.

Yoga Practices for Self-Awareness

In the journey of self-discovery, yoga practices extend beyond poses, fostering self-awareness and revealing our unique gifts, thus nurturing our Inner Shine.

Svadhyaya, a unique aspect of yoga meaning self-study, encourages introspection, deepening our understanding of thoughts, feelings, and actions. This can be as simple as quiet contemplation during Savasana (Corpse Pose), fostering natural insights.

Consider the story of Lisa, a busy entrepreneur. Lisa had a frenetic life, always on the move. Then, she discovered the practice of Svadhyaya during her yoga sessions. In Savasana, she would reflect on her thoughts and emotions, uncovering a talent for creative problem-solving that she had never recognized. This revelation, a spark of her Inner Shine, transformed her approach to her business, leading her to new heights of success.

Mantras, another self-awareness tool, channel the mind into a meditative state. As previously discussed, we can synchronize our breath with mantras. This practice further enhances self-awareness and can be incorporated into poses that we haven't extensively explored, such as Warrior III (Virabhadrasana III). Holding the challenging pose while chanting a mantra helps bring attention to inner strength and balance, potentially revealing physical and mental capacities you weren't aware of before.

Breath awareness is crucial in yoga. As discussed earlier, simply focusing on your breath is a yoga practice in itself. As you move through asanas like Extended Triangle Pose (Utthita Trikonasana) or Camel Pose (Ustrasana), conscious breathing can help you tune into your body's responses, deepening self-awareness.

Furthermore, mindfulness, essential to yoga, serves as a powerful tool for self-discovery. Mindful awareness during practices like Fish Pose (Matsyasana) can unearth hidden character aspects, such as patience or introspection, enhancing your Inner Shine.

These practices, integral to yoga, act as conduits to profound self-awareness, enabling recognition and acceptance of our unique gifts and talents. As you continue your yoga journey, consider how these elements of the practice can guide you towards self-discovery, allowing your Inner Shine to radiate brightly.

Practical Tips: Yoga Practices for Cultivating Presence and Mindfulness

Presence and mindfulness, transformative elements of yoga, are powerful in uncovering our unique gifts and talents—enhancing our Inner Shine. Incorporating these practices into your yoga routine can foster a deep sense of self-awareness, opening the door to self-discovery. Here are some practical tips to help you cultivate presence and mindfulness through yoga.

1. **Begin with Intention:** Prior to your practice, establish a commitment to be present and mindful. A simple affirmation like "I am here, I am present," can serve as a consistent reminder to refocus whenever your mind wanders.
2. **Focus on Sensations, Not Goals:** Instead of striving to achieve a perfect pose, focus on the sensations you experience during the

practice. Feel the stretch, observe the strength of your muscles, and listen to your breath. This approach encourages mindfulness and helps to keep you rooted in the present.

3. **Practice Mindful Transitions:** Be mindful not just in the poses, but also during the transitions. Each movement, each breath can be a moment of mindfulness. For instance, as you transition from Warrior II (Virabhadrasana II) into Extended Side Angle Pose (Utthita Parsvakonasana), pay attention to the shift in your body and breath.

4. **Use Props Mindfully:** Props like blocks, straps, or bolsters can support your practice and enhance your awareness. For example, using a block in Triangle Pose (Trikonasana) can help you focus on alignment and breath, fostering presence and mindfulness.

5. **Practice Mindful Breathing:** Although we've covered breath in-depth in another chapter, it's worth reiterating its importance. Conscious breathing can anchor you in the present moment. Even when not practicing asanas, take a few moments during the day to simply observe your breath.

6. **End with Savasana:** Savasana (Corpse Pose), the final relaxation pose, is an excellent opportunity to practice mindfulness. In the stillness of Savasana, observe your thoughts, feelings, and sensations without judgment. This quiet observation can lead to profound moments of self-discovery.

7. **Incorporate Meditation:** After your yoga practice, take a few minutes to meditate. This can help consolidate the mindfulness cultivated during your practice, allowing you to carry that mindfulness into the rest of your day.

Consider Sarah's story. Sarah, a busy mother of two, was often frazzled and felt she was just surviving each day. When she started incorporating these mindfulness practices into her yoga routine, she noticed a change. She became more present in her daily activities, whether it was making breakfast for her children, working on a project, or practicing yoga. This newfound presence led her to discover a latent talent for painting. As she embraced this talent, she felt a sense of fulfillment and joy that she had never experienced before.

Her Inner Shine began to radiate, touching not just her life, but also the lives of those around her.

Just like Sarah, as you cultivate presence and mindfulness through yoga, you create space for your Inner Shine to emerge. These practices help peel back the layers of distraction and busyness, revealing your unique gifts and talents. Remember, the journey to self-discovery is not always straightforward. It requires patience, perseverance, and a willingness to explore the depths of your inner self. But rest assured, as you continue this journey, you'll find that the rewards are well worth the effort.

Providing Concrete Advice

As we delve deeper into yoga as a tool for cultivating presence, mindfulness, and ultimately revealing our Inner Shine, here are some practical pieces of advice you can incorporate into your daily routine.

- **Consistency is Key:** Commence with a pledge to maintain regular practice. Even a few minutes of daily mindful yoga can make a significant impact.
- **Choose a Quiet Space:** Select a peaceful and comfortable spot in your home where you can practice undisturbed. This environment plays a vital role in creating a serene mindset, which is conducive to mindful practice
- **Tune in to Yourself:** Yoga is an inward journey. Give yourself the freedom to modify poses based on your comfort and capacity. The aim is not to achieve the 'perfect pose', but to listen to your body and respect its limits.
- **Harness the Power of Breath:** We have already discussed the importance of breath in yoga, but it bears repeating. Your breath is the bridge between your body and mind; use it to anchor your attention in the present moment. Remember, the breath is the rhythm of life, tune into it.
- **Take a Moment of Stillness:** After each session, spend a few moments in Savasana, absorbing the effects of your practice. It's a precious opportunity for introspection and to connect with your Inner Shine.

- **Reflect on Your Practice:** As you continue to grow in your yoga journey, remember the value of reflection. As we've discussed in previous chapters, keeping a yoga journal can be a powerful tool for this. After each practice, consider writing your thoughts, feelings, and insights. This can serve as a reminder of your growth and the journey you're on.

- **Embrace Patience:** The journey towards self-discovery and enhancing your Inner Shine is a process, not an event. Be patient with yourself. Celebrate small victories and remember, every step forward, no matter how small, is progress.

Let's consider the case of Mark. He was a high-achieving corporate professional, always racing against time. When he discovered yoga, it was a slow start. But as he incorporated these pieces of advice into his routine, he began to notice a profound shift. He was more mindful, more present in his interactions, and was able to tap into his creative side, a talent he was previously oblivious to. His Inner Shine emerged, and his life transformed.

In essence, the practice of yoga offers you the platform to explore your depths, to understand your unique gifts and talents, and to let your Inner Shine radiate. It's a journey of self-discovery, and these practical tips can serve as your guiding map.

Yoga Poses and Meditation Practices for Mindfulness

Fostering mindfulness through yoga is a voyage of inner exploration. Let's delve into some specific asanas and meditation practices that can help us walk this path, enhancing our awareness and letting our unique gifts and talents shine.

- **Half Moon Pose (Ardha Chandrasana):** This pose demands presence and balance. As you align your body in this posture, it requires mental and physical steadiness, drawing your focus to the present moment. It's not just a physical balancing act but a mental one, too, giving us the opportunity to explore our resilience.

- **Warrior I (Virabhadrasana I):** Grounded and strong, this pose embodies mindful presence. As you root down through your feet and reach up through your hands, there's a sense of anchoring in the present, awakening your inner strength – a crucial aspect of your Inner Shine.

- **Crow Pose (Bakasana):** This arm balance pose might seem challenging, but it's an excellent practice in patience, focus, and overcoming fear – attributes that help in self-discovery and mindful living.
- **Yin Yoga:** This style of yoga involves holding poses for longer periods. It encourages you to slow down, breathe, and stay with your sensations, promoting mindfulness and acceptance.

Now let's turn to meditation practices.

- **Loving-Kindness Meditation (Metta Bhavana):** This meditation cultivates an attitude of goodwill towards ourselves and others. It fosters self-compassion, a key factor in recognizing and accepting our unique gifts and talents.
- **Mindfulness Breathing Meditation:** This practice involves focusing on your breath, observing each inhale and exhale without changing it. This simple yet powerful practice hones your attention and fosters a deep sense of presence.

Take the example of Laura, a busy mother of two, juggling multiple roles. Incorporating these poses and meditation practices into her routine helped her cultivate mindfulness, enabling her to connect with her innate talent for creative problem-solving. This not only helped her manage her daily challenges but also made her recognize her gift, enhancing her Inner Shine.

Remember, these practices are not ends in themselves but tools to guide you on your journey of self-discovery, helping you illuminate your unique gifts and talents. As you continue to explore these practices, may you find your Inner Shine growing ever brighter.

Awakening Inner Strength: A Mindful Yoga Exercise

This 15-minute yoga sequence helps tap into your inner strength and resilience. Remember, adapt the poses to honor your body's limits.

1. Extended Triangle Pose (Utthita Trikonasana)
    - Stand tall at the top of your mat. Step your right foot back about a meter, turning it out to about 60 degrees.

- Extend your arms out to the sides at shoulder height. Reach forward with your left hand and down to your shin or a yoga block. Extend your right arm straight up.
- Hold for 5 breaths, then repeat on the other side.

[Modification: If balance is a challenge, use a wall for support.]

2. Three-Legged Downward-Facing Dog (Tri Pada Adho Mukha Svanasana)
   - From a standing position, bend over and place your hands on the mat. Step both feet back to come into Downward-Facing Dog.
   - Lift your right leg up as high as comfortable, keeping the hips square.
   - Hold for 5 breaths, then repeat with the left leg.

[Modification: If this is too intense, keep both feet on the ground for a regular Downward-Facing Dog.]

3. Half Lord of the Fishes Pose (Ardha Matsyendrasana)
   - Come to a seated position with both legs extended in front of you.
   - Bend your right knee and place your foot outside your left thigh. Bend your left knee, bringing your heel to your right hip.
   - Twist your torso to the right, placing your left elbow outside your right knee for support.
   - Hold for 5 breaths, then repeat on the other side.

[Modification: If the twist is too intense, simply hug your bent knee with your opposite arm.]

4. Savasana (Corpse Pose)
   - Lay on your back, letting your feet fall open. Rest your arms at your sides, palms up.
   - Close your eyes, taking slow deep breaths, surrendering any remaining tension.
   - Stay here for as long as you need.

[Modification: If this causes discomfort in your lower back, bend your knees and plant your feet on the mat.]

This sequence is intended to cultivate inner strength and resilience. With each breath and movement, visualize yourself tapping into your inner well of power, feeling grounded, and capable. Always remember, the journey is yours to navigate, and each practice is a step towards a stronger, more resilient you.

Gently come back to awareness, wiggling your fingers and toes. Roll to one side and press yourself up to a comfortable seated position. Namaste.

Cultivating and Sharing Your Inner Shine: A Radiant Journey

Personal growth is a tapestry of resilience, joy, and challenges. Crucial to this journey is your 'inner shine', your unique blend of talents. This chapter guides you to harness, project, and inspire others with your inner shine A key element in this journey is our "inner shine" – a unique blend of gifts, talents, and attributes. This chapter aims to guide you in harnessing and projecting this inner shine, serving as an inspiration for others on their self-discovery path.

The cultivation of your inner shine commences with self-awareness. Life's fast pace often causes us to lose sight of our unique essence - the distinct gifts and talents we are born with. It's crucial to slow down, align with your authentic self, and recognize the inherent qualities defining you. Whether it's empathy, artistic talent, humor, analytical skills, or quiet strength, these traits contribute to your inner shine.

Embracing your inner shine is a testament to self-love and acceptance. It is about recognizing your unique contributions to the world and appreciating them. It's about letting go of comparison and competition, and instead, stepping into your light with confidence and joy. Remember, the sun doesn't compare with the moon; they both shine when it's their time.

Once you've identified and embraced your inner shine, it's time to share it with the world. Sharing your inner shine is an act of courage and vulnerability. It's about showcasing your authentic self and using your gifts and talents to positively impact those around you. Your inner shine becomes a powerful force of inspiration when shared with others.

Let's imagine you have a talent for storytelling. Sharing this gift might involve writing a heartfelt blog post, recording a podcast, or simply sharing a story with a friend over coffee. Your words might spark inspiration, provide comfort, or evoke a broad smile. The act of sharing your inner shine doesn't have to be grandiose; it simply involves expressing your authentic self in ways that resonate with you.

When you share your inner shine, you inadvertently give others the permission to do the same. You become a living testament to the beauty of authenticity, and this can inspire others to embark on their journey of self-discovery. It's like a ripple effect; your inner shine can inspire others to find and embrace their inner light, creating a cycle of inspiration and growth.

Moreover, sharing your inner shine contributes to your personal fulfillment. There's a profound joy and satisfaction that comes from using your unique gifts and talents in ways that uplift others. It adds a deeper layer of meaning and purpose to your life, further fueling your inner shine.

However, it's important to remember that cultivating and sharing your inner shine is not a one-time event but a continuous process. It requires patience, courage, and self-compassion. There might be days when you feel disconnected from your inner shine, and that's okay. It's all part of the journey. On such days, be gentle with yourself, and remember that your inner shine is still there, waiting for you to rediscover it.

Your inner shine is your unique light in this world. Cultivating and sharing this inner shine not only contributes to your fulfillment but also serves as an inspiration for others. So, embrace your unique gifts, showcase them with pride and love, and watch as you inspire others to do the same, creating a radiant tapestry of shared growth and discovery. Always remember, your inner shine is a gift to the world. Let it glow brightly.

Nurturing Your Inner Shine Through Intention-Setting

Setting intentions plants seeds for nurturing our inner shine. Aligning focus with desires fosters an environment where unique gifts flourish. By aligning our focus with our desires, we foster an environment for our unique gifts and talents to flourish.

Imagine your inner shine as a beautiful, radiant light within you. This light is the essence of who you are, representing your passions, talents, and the distinctive qualities that make you unique. But sometimes, this light may dim or become obscured by the dust of everyday life. This is where the power of intention-setting comes in.

Setting intentions isn't about setting rigid goals or creating a detailed road map for your life. Rather, it's about defining your personal "north star", a guiding beacon that aligns your actions with your innermost desires and values. As you set your intentions, you're consciously choosing to nurture and amplify your inner shine.

Think about what you want your inner shine to represent. Do you wish to radiate kindness, creativity, resilience, or perhaps a blend of all three? Once you identify this, set an intention to live by these qualities. An intention could be as simple as, "I choose to embody kindness in my interactions today," or "I aim to express my creativity in every opportunity I get."

Visualization is a powerful ally in this process. Close your eyes and picture your inner shine as a vibrant light. See it growing brighter as you nurture it with your intentions. Visualize yourself living out these intentions, and observe how it affects your interactions, decisions, and overall sense of well-being.

This practice of intention-setting and visualization serves as a compass, guiding your journey of self-discovery and personal fulfillment. As you align your actions with your intentions daily, you'll notice your inner shine becoming more evident, not just to you, but to everyone around you.

Remember, your inner shine is a beacon that can guide and inspire others. As you nurture it and allow it to radiate brightly, you empower others to embark on their own journey of self-discovery. So, set your intentions, visualize your inner shine, and step forward on your path with confidence and purpose. Your journey to personal fulfillment is just beginning.

Self-Assessment: Identifying Your Unique Gifts

Self-assessment, an introspective process, is key to identifying unique talents. In a world promoting conformity, it's easy to undervalue our abilities. Recognizing and honoring our strengths is the first step towards nurturing our inner shine. In a world that often encourages conformity, it's easy to overlook or undervalue our own abilities. But recognizing and honoring our distinctive strengths is the first step towards nurturing our inner shine. So, how do we undertake this journey of self-discovery? Let's explore a step-by-step guide to conduct a meaningful self-assessment.

Step 1: Self-Reflection

Begin with self-reflection. This is a quiet, introspective exercise, best done in a calm, distraction-free environment. Think about the times when you've felt most alive, most engaged, and most fulfilled. What were you doing? How did it make you feel? Jot down these instances and the skills or qualities they involved. This could range from your ability to listen empathetically, your knack for creative problem-solving, or your aptitude for leadership.

Step 2: Seek Feedback

Next, solicit input from others. Sometimes, we're blind to our own talents, and it takes an outside perspective to bring them into focus. Ask trusted friends, colleagues, or mentors about what they perceive as your strengths. You might be surprised to discover talents you weren't aware of, or have others affirm those you've been uncertain about.

Step 3: Recognize Patterns

With this wealth of information, look for recurring themes. Are there specific talents or strengths that keep showing up? Perhaps you've been complimented on your creative thinking both at work and in your personal life. Or maybe your ability to inspire others has been noted by friends and colleagues alike. These recurring attributes are strong indicators of your unique gifts.

Step 4: Embrace and Value Your Unique Gifts

Once you've identified these gifts, embrace them. This is the heart of your inner shine. It's vital to recognize that your unique abilities are valuable and contribute significantly to the world around you. They set you apart and allow you to make a distinct impact.

Step 5: Utilize Your Gifts

Finally, devise ways to utilize these gifts more effectively in your daily life. This could mean seeking out roles or responsibilities that align with your strengths, or it might involve developing hobbies that allow you to express your unique talents.

Self-assessment is the mirror that reflects our inner shine. It's through this process that we recognize our unique gifts and learn how best to share them with the world. By recognizing, embracing, and utilizing our distinctive strengths, we not only enhance our own sense of fulfillment but also inspire others to embark on their journey of self-discovery.

Remember, your inner shine is not just about what you do well; it's about what you do uniquely well. It's the amalgamation of your talents, experiences, and passions. By identifying these through self-assessment, you're not merely learning about yourself; you're honoring your uniqueness and taking the first step towards a life that's not only successful but also deeply fulfilling.

So take the time for self-assessment, and prepare to be surprised, enlightened, and inspired. As you discover and nurture your unique gifts, you'll find your inner shine growing brighter, guiding you towards a life of authenticity, purpose, and fulfillment.

The Role of Yoga in Connecting with the Present Moment

Yoga provides a unique opportunity to foster a deep connection with the present moment, helping us discover and express our unique gifts and talents. This practice enhances our innate luminescence and allows us to unlock our fullest potential.

"One key aspect of yoga fostering a connection with the present moment is mindfulness—the art of paying attention to our thoughts, emotions, and bodily sensations without judgment. During a yoga practice, we bring our awareness to the breath, the alignment of our bodies, and the sensations we experience in each pose. This focus encourages us to release past or future preoccupations, immersing ourselves fully in the present.

Furthermore, yoga's emphasis on balance and harmony serves to remind us of the importance of maintaining equilibrium in our lives. As we strive to find balance in our bodies, we also learn to find balance in our thoughts and emotions. This sense of harmony fosters a deeper connection with the present moment, allowing us to tap into our unique gifts and augment our inherent glow.

Another way that yoga helps to deepen our connection with the present moment is through the cultivation of non-attachment. In yoga, we learn to let go of our expectations and accept each experience as it is. This practice of non-attachment encourages us to release our grip on the past and the future, freeing us to fully engage with the present moment. As we embrace the present, we become more attuned to our inner shine, allowing it to guide us on our journey of self-discovery.

Yoga's emphasis on balance reminds us of the importance of equilibrium in our lives. Striving for bodily equilibrium helps us attain mental and emotional stability, fostering a deeper connection with the present moment and magnifying our inherent glow.

Yoga offers a powerful avenue for connecting with the present moment, allowing us to discover and express our unique gifts and talents. Through mindfulness, non-attachment, and a focus on balance, yoga helps us to nurture our inner shine, creating a more fulfilling and authentic life experience. By incorporating a consistent yoga practice into our lives, we can cultivate a deeper connection with the present moment, enabling us to fully embrace our innate luminosity and share it with the world.

Enhancing Your Inner Shine Through the Present Moment

Living fully in the present is akin to igniting our inherent glow, freeing us from past regrets and future anxieties, and allowing our unique talents to illuminate our lives.

Mindfulness is the key. By focusing on our breath, the feel of the wind on our skin, the sounds that surround us, we can anchor ourselves in the present. Each moment is a canvas, and mindfulness is the brush that lets us paint with the vibrant colors of our gifts and talents.

Being present allows us to heed the whispers of our intuition, steering us towards our passion and purpose. This connection with the present moment frees us from distractions, allowing us to fully engage with our tasks, ideas, and people around us. The more present we are, the more our inner shine radiates, revealing our unique gifts.

In essence, embracing the present moment enables us to live mindfully, attuning to our gifts and letting our inner shine guide us towards an authentic and fulfilling life.

Guided Visualization Exercise: Imagining Your Future Self

Close your eyes, and let's embark on a journey to meet your future self, the version of you who has fully embraced their inner shine.

Imagine yourself in a serene, peaceful place. It could be a lush forest, a tranquil beach, or a cozy room. This is your safe haven, a place where you can be completely at ease.

Now, visualize a path extending from where you stand. The path represents your journey forward in life. Begin walking along this path, feeling anticipation and excitement bubbling within you.

As you stroll, you see a figure in the distance. This figure radiates a comforting, warm light - this is your future self, the embodiment of your fully realized potential.

Approach your future self, take note of how confident and content they appear. They're the living representation of your inner shine, your unique gifts and talents expressed freely. How do they interact with the world around them? What actions are they taking that reflect their inner shine?

Now, your future self turns to you and shares a piece of wisdom, a key to unlocking your inner shine. Listen carefully. This message is something you can start implementing in your life today to nurture your gifts and talents.

Take a moment to absorb this wisdom. Feel a sense of gratitude towards your future self for this insight. Know that this future self is not a distant dream, but a reality that you're in the process of creating.

Slowly bring your awareness back to the present. Open your eyes. Hold onto the vision of your future self, let it motivate you to embrace your inner shine, and guide you in setting intentions that align with expressing your unique gifts and talents. Remember, this journey is yours, and every step you take brings you closer to your illuminated self.

Concluding Meditation: Embracing Your Unique Gifts and Talents

As we conclude, let's enter a space of quiet reflection with a meditation focused on embracing our unique gifts and talents.

Settle into a comfortable position. Allow your body to relax and your mind to calm. Close your eyes, inhale deeply, and as you exhale, let go of any tension you may be holding.

Visualize a radiant light glowing within your heart—your inherent glow, the authentic expression of your unique talents.

Now, imagine this light expanding with each breath you take, filling every inch of your being, illuminating your gifts and talents. Let it shine so brightly that it overflows, extending outward into the world around you.

As you sit with this luminous energy, think about your unique gifts and talents. How do they enrich your life? How do they impact the world around you? Allow yourself to feel a deep sense of appreciation for these unique aspects of yourself.

Now, set an intention to honor your inner shine in your daily life. Envision yourself living in alignment with your gifts, sharing them freely and joyfully. Feel the deep fulfillment that comes from this alignment.

Take a moment to bask in this feeling of fulfillment. Allow it to embed itself deeply within you, serving as a guidepost on your journey of self-discovery and personal fulfillment.

As we come to the end of this meditation, gently bring your awareness back to your surroundings. Open your eyes, carrying with you the image of your radiant inner shine and the commitment to honor your unique gifts and talents.

Your inherent glow serves as a beacon of inspiration and guidance. Embrace and nurture it, letting it illuminate your path towards a fulfilled existence.

7

Yoga for Emotional Healing: Nurturing Your Inner Self through Yoga

As we venture further into our journey, we now turn our focus towards the power of yoga as a tool for emotional healing. It's one thing to bask in our inner shine, as we did in our previous chapter, but how do we sustain that radiance when emotional clouds darken our skies? The beauty of yoga lies in its inherent ability to cleanse, heal, and renew, not just our physical bodies, but our emotional selves as well.

Like you, my journey through yoga hasn't been solely physical. I've discovered yoga as a sanctuary, a place to retreat when my emotions seem overwhelming. Let me share a personal anecdote.

A few years back, I experienced a significant upheaval in my life. The emotional turmoil was overwhelming, a wave that threatened to pull me under. In the midst of this emotional storm, I turned to my yoga mat.

It wasn't about performing the most complex asanas, but rather about connecting with myself on a deeper level. The simple act of focusing on my breath, of feeling the ebb and flow of my life force, brought me back to the present moment. Each pose became an act of self-care, a message of love and support to my heavy heart.

One day, as I was gently flowing through a sequence, tears started to roll down my cheeks. I realized that I wasn't just moving my body; I was moving my distress. With each breath, each movement, I was letting go, not of the profound connection I felt for what I had lost, but of the pain that had lodged itself in my heart.

The journey was not instantaneous. Healing never is. But with time, yoga became my lifeline. It taught me to nurture my inner self, to honor my feelings, and to find peace in the present moment, no matter how tumultuous the sea of emotions might be."

As we delve into this chapter, we'll explore how yoga can be a potent tool in our emotional healing journey. We'll look at specific practices designed to help us manage stress, release emotional blockages, and foster a deep sense of inner peace. This is a journey into the soul of yoga, where the mat serves as a mirror, reflecting our inner selves back to us.

As we face our emotions bravely, let's remember to carry our radiant inner shine with us. It is our guide, our beacon, as we navigate the path towards emotional healing and wholeness.

The Connection between Yoga and Emotional Healing

In the vast expanse of yoga, we find an inherent connection between our physical practices and emotional well-being. Yoga is not just about flexibility or strength; it is a holistic journey of self-discovery, healing, and transformation. As we peel back the layers, we come to understand how deeply yoga intertwines with our emotional health.

Historical Background of Yoga for Emotional Healing

Yoga, from its inception, has been a holistic practice, encompassing not just the physical, but the mental and emotional spheres as well. The ancient yogis believed in the deep interconnectedness of mind and body. They understood that emotional upheavals could translate into physical discomfort, and conversely, physical ailments could stem from emotional distress. Thus, the practice of yoga was devised to bring about equilibrium in body and mind.

The foundational text, the "Yoga Sutras of Patanjali," underscores the principle of emotional well-being. Patanjali, the revered sage, defined yoga as the calming of the mind's fluctuations. In this tranquil state, we encounter clarity, peace, and the opportunity for healing. While the physical poses we associate with yoga today were not detailed in Patanjali's Sutras, the philosophical essence deeply aligns with emotional healing.

Philosophical Aspects of Yoga and Emotional Healing

As we explore the philosophy of yoga, we encounter several principles that bolster emotional healing. One such principle is 'Ahimsa,' meaning non-violence. Ahimsa invites us to show kindness and compassion towards all beings, including ourselves. Much of our emotional distress springs from a deficit of self-love. Through Ahimsa, we learn to treat ourselves with kindness, which becomes a catalyst for emotional healing.

Apart from Ahimsa, the philosophy of yoga also emphasizes 'Santosha,' or contentment. Santosha teaches us to find peace in our current circumstances, regardless of what they may be. This acceptance can help us manage emotional upheaval, leading to a state of inner peace and tranquility.

Practical Tip: Integrating Yoga Philosophy into Daily Life

So how can you bring these philosophical tenets into your everyday life? The answer is surprisingly straightforward. Begin by carving out moments of quietude in your day. This could be a mere five minutes of sitting in silence, focusing on your breath. These tranquil moments can provide insight into your emotional state, promoting self-awareness.

Practicing Ahimsa starts with the words you employ when conversing with yourself. Are they critical and judgmental or compassionate and understanding? When you detect negative self-talk, gently steer your thoughts towards kindness and empathy. This act of self-love can have a profound influence on your emotional well-being.

Incorporating yoga philosophy into your life doesn't necessitate hours spent on the yoga mat. It's about subtle shifts in your perspective, gentle reminders of self-awareness, self-love, and mindfulness. As you traverse your day embodying the principles of yoga, you may notice a change, a softening in your emotional landscape. It's in this subtle transformation that you truly encounter the healing power of yoga.

The Benefits of Practicing Yoga for Emotional Well-being

Stepping onto your yoga mat, you enter a sacred space. A space where you can let go of external demands and turn your focus inward. In this safe haven, you have the opportunity to reconnect with yourself on a deeper level, a journey that extends beyond mere physical wellness and ventures into the realm of emotional well-being.

Yoga, in its essence, is a practice of unity. It binds the body, mind, and spirit in a harmonious dance, each movement echoing with potential for healing. When we face emotional turbulence, this practice of integration can become our solace, our guiding light amidst the storm. The benefits of yoga for emotional well-being are both profound and multifaceted.

- **Reducing Stress:** Yoga, through its combination of physical postures, breathwork, and meditation, has been found to lower stress levels. When we're stressed, our bodies go into 'fight or flight' mode, a state that's far from conducive to emotional health. Yoga helps us shift to a 'rest and digest' mode, soothing our nervous system and fostering a sense of calm.
- **Enhancing Emotional Resilience:** Emotional resilience is our ability to cope with life's challenges, to ride the waves of adversity without losing our balance. Yoga strengthens our emotional resilience by teaching us to stay present, to breathe through discomfort, and to approach our experiences with an attitude of non-judgment.
- **Promoting Self-Love:** As we've discussed, principles like Ahimsa and Santosha foster self-compassion and contentment. Regular yoga practice helps us internalize these concepts, leading to a greater sense of self-love and acceptance.
- **Improving Mood and Energy:** The physical aspect of yoga can stimulate the release of 'feel-good' hormones like endorphins. Regular practice can help improve mood, energy levels, and overall outlook on life.

Now, let me share a personal experience. I recall a period in my life when my emotional world felt like a tempest. Amidst this emotional whirlwind, I found solace in my yoga practice. The simple act of stepping onto my mat, of honoring where I was in that moment without pushing or judging, became a source of comfort. As I moved and breathed, I could feel a subtle shift, a lightening of the emotional weight I'd been carrying. It wasn't a quick fix, but over time, yoga became my sanctuary, a space where I could heal and grow.

As you step onto your mat, remember that yoga is not a competition. It's a personal journey, one that honors your unique rhythm and pace. Some days, your practice might be dynamic and energetic. Other days, it might be gentle and restorative. Whatever shape your practice takes, know that each breath, each pose, is a step towards greater emotional well-being.

In the following sections, we'll explore specific yoga practices that can support emotional healing. You're not alone on this journey. Together, we'll navigate this path, finding strength, resilience, and healing in the transformative power of yoga.

Breathwork Techniques for Emotional Regulation and Balance

Breath is our life force, our connection to the present moment. In yoga, the art of breath control is known as Pranayama, a tool that can guide us towards emotional equilibrium.

Explanation of Pranayama

Pranayama is a Sanskrit term where 'Prana' means life force or vital energy and 'Ayama' means control or expansion. Through Pranayama, we learn to harness the power of our breath, using it as a bridge between the mind and body. This connection can play a pivotal role in regulating our emotions, helping us cultivate a balanced mental state.

Techniques for Emotional Regulation

There are several Pranayama techniques that can aid in emotional regulation. Let's explore a couple:1.

1. **Nadi Shodhana** (Alternate Nostril Breathing): This technique promotes balance by harmonizing the left and right hemispheres of the brain. It induces calm and reduces anxiety, making it an excellent tool for emotional regulation.
2. **Bhramari Pranayama** (Bee Breath): The humming sound produced during Bee Breath soothes the nervous system and calms the mind, making it beneficial for those dealing with emotional distress.

Step-by-Step Instructions for Practice

Nadi Shodhana:

1. Sit comfortably with your spine erect.
2. Close your eyes and take a few deep breaths.
3. Close your right nostril with your right thumb and inhale slowly through your left nostril.
4. Close your left nostril with your ring finger, open your right nostril, and exhale slowly.
5. Keeping the left nostril closed, inhale through the right nostril. Then close the right nostril and exhale through the left. This completes one round.
6. Continue for 5-10 rounds, then return to normal breathing and observe the effects.

Bhramari Pranayama:

1. Sit comfortably with your spine erect.
2. Close your eyes and take a few deep breaths.
3. Close your ears with your thumbs and place your fingers gently over your eyes.
4. Inhale deeply, then exhale slowly while making a humming sound like a bee.
5. Repeat 5-10 times, then return to normal breathing and observe the effects.

Guided Breathwork Meditation for Emotional Balance

Close your eyes and sit comfortably. Take a moment to scan your body, releasing any tension. Now, bring your attention to your breath. Don't try to change it, just observe.

Imagine your breath as a gentle wave, washing over you with each inhale and receding with each exhale. Feel the rhythm, the ebb, and flow. Now, let's transition into Nadi Shodhana. Follow the steps provided earlier, allowing your breath to guide you towards balance.

After a few rounds, let's shift into Bhramari Pranayama. As you make the humming sound, imagine it vibrating through your body, soothing your nerves, calming your mind.

After your final round, return to normal breathing. Sit in silence for a few moments, absorbing the effects of your practice. When you're ready, gently open your eyes.

Remember, your breath is always with you, a beacon of calm amidst the storm of emotions. Through these Pranayama techniques, you can tap into the power of your breath, cultivating emotional balance and wellbeing. So next time you feel the waves of emotions rising, pause, breathe, and find your center.

The Role of Mindfulness in Yoga for Emotional Healing

Mindfulness, a concept that has become synonymous with yoga and meditation, holds significant potential in our quest for emotional healing.

Understanding Mindfulness

Mindfulness refers to the practice of being fully present in the moment, of observing our thoughts, emotions, and sensations without judgment. It invites us to step back from the constant chatter of the mind, offering a space for clarity and insight.

Mindfulness in Yoga

In yoga, mindfulness takes center stage. With each breath, each asana, we are encouraged to stay present. Notice the sensation of your foot grounding into the mat in Mountain Pose (Tadasana), the gentle expansion of your chest as you breathe in Child's Pose (Balasana). This conscious attention brings depth to our practice, transforming it from a mere physical exercise into a journey of self-discovery.

Mindfulness and Emotional Healing

When we apply mindfulness to our emotional landscape, it opens the door to healing. By observing our emotions without getting caught in the storyline, we can recognize them as transient states, not defining traits. This shift in perspective can alleviate emotional distress, fostering resilience and well-being.

Consider a time when you felt overwhelmed by emotions. Perhaps you were anxious about a presentation or frustrated with a friend. Now, imagine observing these emotions as a bystander, acknowledging their presence without judgment or resistance. Suddenly, their hold over you softens. This is the power of mindfulness in emotional healing.

Reflect on your experiences of mindfulness in your yoga practice. Have there been moments when you felt fully present, completely absorbed in the sensation of a pose or the rhythm of your breath? How did this affect your emotional state?

Reflecting on these experiences can deepen our understanding of mindfulness, enabling us to integrate it into our daily lives. As we navigate the ebbs and flows of our emotions, mindfulness serves as an anchor, rooting us in the present and guiding us towards healing.

Remember, mindfulness, like yoga, is a practice. It's not about perfection but progress. So, as you step onto your mat, invite mindfulness to join you. Embrace the journey with an open heart, knowing that with each mindful breath, each mindful movement, you're nurturing your emotional well-being. Yoga is not just a practice but a path to self-discovery, emotional healing, and inner peace. So, keep practicing, keep exploring, and let the transformative power of yoga guide you towards emotional balance and serenity.

Incorporating Meditation into Your Yoga Practice for Emotional Well-being

Meditation, an integral part of the yoga tradition, offers profound benefits for emotional well-being. It provides us the opportunity to quiet the mind and connect with our inner selves on a deeper level.

Importance of Meditation in Yoga

Within the intricate mosaic of yoga, meditation is like the golden thread that binds it all together. It takes us beyond the physical, into the realm of the mind and spirit. The asanas prepare our bodies for meditation, while pranayama paves the way for a calm and focused mind.

Effects on Emotional Health

Meditation invites us to observe our thoughts and emotions without judgment, fostering self-awareness and acceptance. It helps us break free from the cycle of negative thinking, and over time, can cultivate emotional resilience. By connecting with our inner selves, we gain insight into our emotional patterns, empowering us to navigate life's ups and downs with grace and equanimity.

Guide to Integrating Meditation

Integrating meditation into your yoga routine can be as simple as dedicating a few minutes at the end of your practice to sit in silence. Here's a basic guide:

1. After completing your asanas and pranayama, find a comfortable seated position.
2. Close your eyes and bring your attention to your breath. Don't try to control it, just observe.
3. If your mind wanders, gently bring it back to the breath. Remember, the goal is not to empty the mind, but to become aware of your thoughts without getting caught up in them.
4. Start with just a few minutes and gradually increase the duration as your comfort level grows.

Practical Tip: Consistency is key in meditation. Try to meditate at the same time each day, creating a ritual that signals to your mind that it's time to quiet down. Even on days when sitting still feels like a challenge, commit to a few minutes. This consistency can create a momentum that carries your practice forward.

Remember, meditation is a journey, not a destination. There will be days when it feels effortless, and days when it feels like a struggle. But every moment you spend in meditation is a step towards greater emotional well-being. So, as you roll out your yoga mat, remember to make space for meditation. It's in this silence that we often find our greatest insights, our deepest healing. In the quietude of meditation, we can nurture our inner selves, fostering emotional balance and tranquility.

Yoga Practices for Healing Emotional Wounds

Yoga, with its myriad of poses and practices, can serve as a healing balm for emotional wounds. Certain postures, in particular, can create a space for emotional release, fostering a sense of peace and well-being.

Overview of Healing Practices

While we've explored many asanas in this journey, there are a few postures particularly conducive to emotional healing. Two such poses are the Extended Puppy Pose (Uttana Shishosana) and the Reclining Bound Angle Pose (Supta Baddha Konasana).

Extended Puppy Pose, a heart-opening posture, can help release pent-up emotions, while Reclining Bound Angle Pose encourages a deep sense of relaxation and surrender, nurturing emotional healing.

Effects of these Practices

Extended Puppy Pose gently stretches the spine and shoulders, promoting relaxation and reducing stress. By opening the heart area, this pose invites emotional release, helping us let go of emotional pain.

Reclining Bound Angle Pose, on the other hand, stimulates the heart and improves circulation, promoting a sense of calm and well-being. It opens the hips, often regarded as the seat of our emotions, helping to release emotional tension.

Let's walk through a healing sequence incorporating these postures.

1. Extended Puppy Pose (Uttana Shishosana)

    • Begin on all fours, with your shoulders over your wrists and your hips over your knees.

    • Walk your hands forward, lowering your chest towards the ground. Keep your hips over your knees and your arms shoulder-width apart.

    • Rest your forehead on the mat, feeling a gentle stretch in your spine and shoulders.

    • Breathe deeply and hold for 5-10 breaths.

2. Reclining Bound Angle Pose (Supta Baddha Konasana)

    • From a seated position, bring the soles of your feet together, allowing your knees to fall out to the sides.

- Slowly lean back onto your hands, then onto your forearms and finally, lay your back on the ground.

- Place your hands on your lower belly or let your arms fall to the sides, palms up.

- Relax and breathe deeply, holding for 5-10 breaths.

As you move through this sequence, allow your breath to guide you, creating space for any emotions that may arise. Remember, it's okay to feel. Release any judgment and let the healing energy of yoga do its work.

End your practice with a few moments of quiet reflection in Savasana, noticing any shifts in your emotional state. This sequence can be a gentle step towards healing emotional wounds, cultivating a deeper connection with your inner self, and moving towards emotional well-being. As always, listen to your body and modify as needed. Trust the process, trust the journey.

Specific Yoga Sequences for Different Emotional States (e.g., Anxiety, Depression, Anger)

Life can sometimes throw curveballs, and our emotional states might fluctuate. In this chapter, we'll explore specific yoga sequences to support you during periods of anxiety, depression, and anger. I'll guide you on how and when to use these sequences, and we'll include a self-assessment quiz to help you identify your emotional state and the most suitable yoga sequence for your needs.

Yoga for Anxiety

Anxiety can feel overwhelming, and finding ways to manage it is essential. This calming yoga sequence is designed to help ground and center you, promoting a sense of relaxation and tranquility.

1. Easy Pose (Sukhasana) with Deep Breathing - 3 minutes
2. Cat-Cow Pose (Marjaryasana-Bitilasana) - 5 breaths
3. Child's Pose (Balasana) - 10 breaths
4. Legs Up the Wall (Viparita Karani) - 3 minutes
5. Seated Forward Bend (Paschimottanasana) - 5 breaths

6. Corpse Pose (Savasana) - 5 minutes

Yoga for Depression

Depression can weigh you down, leaving you feeling drained and disinterested. This invigorating yoga sequence aims to uplift your energy and mood, fostering a sense of hope and resilience.

1. Mountain Pose (Tadasana) - 5 breaths
2. Sun Salutations (Surya Namaskar) - 3 rounds
3. Warrior I (Virabhadrasana I) - 5 breaths each side
4. Triangle Pose (Utthita Trikonasana) - 5 breaths each side
5. Camel Pose (Ustrasana) - 5 breaths
6. Fish Pose (Matsyasana) - 5 breaths
7. Corpse Pose (Savasana) - 5 minutes

Yoga for Anger

Anger can be consuming, and finding healthy ways to release it is crucial. This grounding and centering yoga sequence is designed to help you process your emotions and cultivate inner peace.

1. Seated Twist (Ardha Matsyendrasana) - 5 breaths each side
2. Eagle Pose (Garudasana) - 5 breaths each side
3. Forward Fold (Uttanasana) - 5 breaths
4. Pigeon Pose (Eka Pada Rajakapotasana) - 5 breaths each side
5. Lion's Breath (Simhasana) - 3 rounds
6. Supine Twist (Supta Matsyendrasana) - 5 breaths each side
7. Corpse Pose (Savasana) - 5 minutes

Self-Assessment Quiz

To help you determine which sequence is best suited for your current emotional state, take a moment to reflect on how you feel. Then, select the sequence that resonates with you the most and follow the steps provided.

1. How do you generally feel when you wake up in the morning?

    A. Refreshed and eager to start the day

B. Anxious about the tasks ahead

C. Depressed and lacking energy

D. Restless and wishing for more sleep

2. Which statement best describes your current emotional state?

    A. I am generally content and at peace

    B. I often feel stressed or overwhelmed

    C. I regularly experience low mood or sadness

    D. I have difficulty calming my mind and relaxing

3. How often do you experience physical tension or pain (e.g., headaches, backaches)?

    A. Rarely

    B. Occasionally, especially during stressful periods

    C. Often, even without identifiable stress

    D. Almost always

4. How would you describe your current relationship with your emotions?

    A. I am in touch with my emotions and can express them healthily

    B. I struggle with certain emotions, especially stress and anxiety

    C. I often feel numb or disconnected from my emotions

    D. My emotions feel overwhelming and hard to manage

5. When you encounter a challenging situation, how do you typically respond?

    A. I approach it calmly and rationally

    B. I become anxious and worried

    C. I feel down and struggle to find a solution

    D. My mind races, and I struggle to focus

Depending on the responses:

Mostly As: You are generally in a balanced emotional state. Choose a yoga sequence that helps maintain this balance and promotes overall well-being.

Mostly Bs: You may be dealing with some stress or anxiety. Opt for a yoga sequence designed to relieve stress and promote relaxation.

Mostly Cs: You may be experiencing low mood or emotional disconnection. Choose a yoga sequence that promotes emotional connection and uplifts mood.

Mostly Ds: You seem to struggle with high anxiety and restlessness. Choose a yoga sequence specifically designed to calm the mind and body.

Remember, yoga is a personal journey, and it's essential to listen to your body and adapt the sequences as needed. As you practice these sequences, you'll discover new ways to connect with your emotions, allowing you to navigate life's challenges with grace and resilience.

Guided Yoga Nidra Session for Emotional Healing

In Chapter 1, we dived into the world of Yoga Nidra, a profound practice that escorts us into the deepest layers of our subconscious while our bodies relax and surrender. Akin to a ferryman guiding us across the river of the mind, Yoga Nidra eases us into profound relaxation, disentangles us from stress, enhances our sleep, unblocks emotional barricades, and taps into our creativity. Among these benefits, we're focusing today on the remarkable capacity of Yoga Nidra for emotional healing.

Guided Yoga Nidra Session

Close your eyes and let my voice guide you. Envision yourself in a peaceful meadow, the sunlight gentle, the breeze soft. As you inhale, allow your body to fill with tranquility, and as you exhale, release any tension you feel.

Feel the support of the Earth beneath you and permit your body to melt into this support. I invite you now to set an intention for this session - a sankalpa - a positive affirmation in the present tense that focuses on emotional healing. Repeat this sankalpa to yourself three times, embedding it deep within your consciousness.

Slowly guide your awareness through your body, starting from the crown of your head, moving down to your toes. As you mentally scan each part, release any stored emotions, envision them as colors, or sensations, evaporating into the air, leaving you lighter.

Now, imagine a healing light, perhaps a warm gold or soothing blue, slowly enveloping you, seeping into every cell, each fiber of your being. Let it guide you towards acceptance, compassion, and love for yourself.

As we come to the end of this short journey, remind yourself of your sankalpa once more, embedding it deeper into your subconscious. When you're ready, slowly bring your awareness back to the physical realm and open your eyes, carrying this feeling of lightness and peace with you throughout your day.

Practical tip: Creating a Serene Environment

To fully immerse yourself in Yoga Nidra, curate a serene environment at home. Choose a space where you feel safe and calm, free from interruptions. Dim the lights or light a few candles, play soft, ambient sounds, perhaps the murmur of a brook or the rustle of leaves. Use a comfortable mat and cover yourself with a light blanket. Remember, the key is to make this space your sanctuary, a place where you feel protected and free to explore your inner world.

Remember, Yoga Nidra is your intimate journey into self-discovery and healing. Trust the process and let the voyage unfold.

The Benefits of Practicing Yoga in Nature for Emotional Healing

Benefits of Outdoor Yoga

There's a peculiar magic in practicing yoga outdoors, a synergy of energies that elevates the experience to an entirely new level. Imagine the soft murmur of leaves, the gentle hum of life all around, the sun's warmth on your skin – it's yoga, but with an enchanting twist.

Outdoor yoga allows us to root ourselves literally in nature, our bodies aligning with the rhythm of the Earth. As we inhale the fresh air, our lungs expand, soaking up the purity, and with each exhale, we release not just carbon dioxide, but the shackles of our anxieties and worries.

The freedom of an open sky encourages flexibility in our minds as well as our bodies. The vastness inspires a shift in perspective, a reminder of the grand scheme of things, and suddenly, our problems seem a little less daunting.

Nature and Emotional Healing

Nature, in all its unassuming beauty, plays a remarkable role in our emotional healing. It's no coincidence that we find peace in the whisper of the wind or the rustle of leaves. Nature, with its infinite wisdom, nurtures, heals, and rejuvenates.

When we immerse ourselves in nature during our yoga practice, we're not just doing asanas, we're engaging in a dialogue with the Earth. As we root our feet into the soil, we draw strength from its steadfastness. As we stretch towards the sky, we embrace its limitlessness. Each pose, each breath, becomes a silent prayer, an intimate exchange of love and gratitude.

Outdoor yoga deepens our connectivity to the universe, making us aware of the life pulsating within and around us. This profound connection amplifies the healing power of yoga, washing over our emotional wounds, gently nudging us towards acceptance, release, and ultimately, healing.

Practical Tip: Finding Your Outdoor Yoga Space

Now you might be thinking, "Where can I practice yoga outdoors?" The answer is simpler than you might imagine. Your ideal yoga space could be your backyard, a nearby park, or even a quiet beach. The goal is to find a place where you feel at ease, surrounded by the calming serenity of nature.

Make sure the ground is flat and safe for practice. Carry a yoga mat or a blanket to ensure comfort. Don't forget to check the weather, and dress appropriately - layers are your friend. And remember, this is your sacred space, so leave your electronic devices behind. Embrace this time as a chance to disconnect from the digital world and reconnect with nature and yourself.

Remember, as you step onto your mat, let nature be your guide. Let the wind remind you to breathe, the trees to stand tall, the rivers to flow freely, and the vast sky to dream without limits. Let nature's symphony accompany your yoga practice, and soon, you'll find your body, mind, and spirit swaying to its harmonious tune, dancing towards emotional healing

Affirmations and Mantras for Emotional Healing

Understanding Affirmations and Mantras

Imagine you're nurturing a seed in your hand. It's small, but holds immense potential within. The words we speak are like these seeds, their power often underestimated. This is where affirmations and mantras, two powerful tools in yoga, come in. They are the water and sunlight, coaxing the seed to sprout, to grow.

Affirmations are positive, empowering statements we say to ourselves, guiding our thoughts and emotions towards healing. Mantras, on the other hand, are sacred phrases often chanted in Sanskrit, carrying profound spiritual energy. Both tools serve the same purpose - to redirect our energy towards positivity, strength, and healing.

Examples for Emotional Healing

Let's explore some affirmations and mantras that can serve as your compass in the journey of emotional healing.

- **Affirmation:** "I am at peace with my past. I welcome the present with love. I am hopeful for my future."
- **Mantra:** "Om Shanti Shanti Shanti" - invoking peace in mind, body, and spirit.
- **Affirmation:** "I forgive myself and others. I release all hurt and embrace healing."
- **Mantra:** "Lokah Samastah Sukhino Bhavantu" - May all beings everywhere be happy and free.

Your Personal Affirmations and Mantras

Now, I invite you to create your own affirmations and mantras. This is a personal journey, and the words you choose should resonate with your heart. Reflect on what you seek - is it peace, forgiveness, strength, love? Craft an affirmation around it. As for mantras, you can pick a Sanskrit phrase that resonates with you or even create a meaningful phrase in your own language.

Remember, these words are seeds. As you repeat them, believe in them, and let them grow within you. With time, you'll find them blossoming into beautiful flowers of healing, transforming your emotional landscape.

Conclusion Embracing Nature and Self for Emotional Healing

As we've journeyed through this chapter, we've discovered the power of blending two of life's most transformative forces: yoga and nature. Their synergy creates an empowering platform for emotional healing, providing a unique way to reconnect with ourselves and the world around us.

Practicing yoga outdoors allows us to root ourselves in nature's rhythm, creating a dialogue with the Earth through each pose and breath. This connection amplifies yoga's healing power, encouraging acceptance, release, and ultimately, emotional healing. But it's not just about the physical asanas; it's about immersing ourselves in the entire experience, from the whisper of the wind to the steadfastness of the soil beneath us.

We also delved into the power of affirmations and mantras, the spoken seeds of healing. Whether they're personal statements of empowerment or sacred Sanskrit phrases, these words hold the potential to redirect our energy towards positivity, strength, and healing.

Your journey to emotional healing is as unique as you are, and there is no one-size-fits-all solution. But by embracing the serenity of nature and the wisdom of yoga, you're taking a monumental step towards a more balanced, peaceful existence.

So, as you unroll your mat under the open sky next time, remember: you are not just practicing yoga; you're embarking on a profound journey of self-discovery and healing. Let the wind remind you to breathe, the trees to stand tall, and the sky to dream limitlessly. Say your affirmations and mantras with conviction, letting them nurture your emotional landscape.

In the words of the ancient yogis, "Lokah Samastah Sukhino Bhavantu" - May all beings everywhere be happy and free. May your journey through yoga in nature bring you the emotional healing you seek, one breath, one pose, and one affirmation at a time

8
Yoga Philosophy for Cultivating Inner Light (Part 1)

As we stepped off the yoga mat in the previous chapter, you learned to harness the healing power of yoga for emotional well-being. Now, let's delve deeper into the labyrinth of yoga philosophy - a fascinating world that extends far beyond the physical postures. Our journey today leads us to the concept of "Inner Light" - a brilliant beacon of self-awareness and truth that yogic philosophy urges us to uncover within ourselves. This path won't be an easy one. Like learning a new language, it's full of strange words and complex concepts. But with patience and openness, we'll make sense of it together.

Understanding the Inner Light

In Yogic philosophy, "Inner Light" refers to our true nature, a state of pure consciousness and self-awareness that's unclouded by external influences or internal turmoil. This inner light, or divine essence, exists within all of us, waiting to be discovered and nurtured. Remember the first time you stood tall in the Tadasana, or Mountain Pose, and felt a profound sense of stillness and strength? That was a glimpse of your inner light. And that's exactly what we aim to cultivate in this chapter.

Self-Assessment: Unveiling your Inner Light

Before we delve further, let's pause for a brief self-assessment. This will help us understand your current perception of Yogic philosophy and the concept of inner light.

1. What does "Inner Light" mean to you?
2. Have you experienced moments of inner light in your yoga practice or otherwise?
3. What are some of the obstacles that dim your inner light?

Don't worry about getting the "right" answers. The purpose of this exercise is to observe your current understanding and feelings towards these concepts. In the upcoming sections, we'll illuminate the Yogic philosophy in a way that will bring a new perspective to these questions.

Cultivating Your Inner Light: The Yogic Path

To nurture our inner light, we delve into the ancient wisdom of Yoga. Its philosophy offers practical guidance on how to cultivate our inner light through practices such as meditation, ethical living, and self-inquiry. But, how do we make these age-old teachings relevant to our modern lives? The answer is simple - by applying them mindfully in our everyday actions and decisions.

As we embark on this exploration, remember: the journey to self-discovery is not a race. It's a continual process of learning and unlearning, shedding light on the corners of our self we've overlooked. So, let's continue this journey with curiosity and openness, eager to embrace the wisdom that awaits us. Together, let's light the path ahead.

Understanding the Yogic Philosophy of Inner Light

In the ancient scriptures of Yoga, "Inner Light," also known as "Jyoti" in Sanskrit, symbolizes the purest form of consciousness, a beacon of self-awareness and truth within us. This concept originates from the Upanishads, the philosophical part of the Vedas, which are the oldest known yoga scriptures. They propound that this light is not just metaphorical; it represents our true nature - unchanging, eternal, and inherently blissful.

Imagine a mountain lake on a calm day, its surface perfectly mirroring the clear sky above. Our mind is like that lake - when it's calm and serene, it reflects the inner light with complete clarity. However, our daily stressors, anxieties, and distractions create ripples on this surface, distorting our reflection of the inner light.

The Inner Light and Your Yoga Practice

So, how does this philosophical concept translate into our yoga practice? Yoga, in its holistic sense, is not just about perfecting the postures. It's about clearing those ripples to perceive our inner light clearly, a state Yogis refer to as "Self-Realization."

Every time you find stillness in a pose, focus your attention in meditation, or find balance in your breath, you are chipping away at the distortions, creating space for your inner light to shine through. This recognition of our true self can profoundly affect our self-awareness and personal growth, allowing us to act with more compassion, integrity, and mindfulness, both on and off the mat.

Cultivating Your Inner Light: An Ongoing Journey

Cultivating inner light is not an overnight transformation; it's an ongoing journey, a gradual process of discovery and growth. It's about becoming more attuned to yourself, recognizing your strengths, acknowledging your limitations, and learning to navigate life with a balanced perspective.

Recommended Readings and Reflection

For a deeper understanding of the yogic philosophy, consider reading the classic texts such as the Upanishads, Bhagavad Gita, and Patanjali's Yoga Sutras. Many contemporary books and online resources also offer simplified interpretations of these ancient texts, making them more accessible to the modern reader.

To further reflect on your understanding of the inner light, consider the following questions:

1. How have you experienced your inner light in your yoga practice?
2. What steps can you take to cultivate your inner light?
3. How might recognizing your inner light influence your daily life?

Remember, there are no right or wrong answers here. These reflections are for you to introspect and gain deeper insights into your personal yoga journey.

As we delve deeper into this concept, let this understanding of the Inner Light illuminate your path, guiding your steps towards greater self-awareness, and ultimately, self-realization. And just as you would with any yoga pose, approach this journey with patience, compassion, and a sense of curiosity, knowing that every step you take is a step closer to your true self.

Applying the Yamas and Niyamas to Your Practice - Yamas and Niyamas: The Ethical Pillars of Yoga

In the vast expanse of yoga philosophy, two cornerstones that stand as guides to enhance our inner light are Yamas and Niyamas. They form the first two limbs of Patanjali's Eightfold Path, offering ethical principles that extend yoga beyond the mat and into our daily lives. Let's embark on an exploration of each of these principles, unveiling their potential to guide us towards our true selves.

Yamas: The Five Moral Restraints

Yamas are the moral, ethical, and societal guidelines for the practicing yogi. They guide us in our interactions with others and the world around us.

1. Ahimsa (Non-violence): Ahimsa teaches us to act with kindness and compassion, not just towards others, but also towards ourselves. For example, recognizing negative self-talk and replacing it with a more nurturing voice can be a practice of Ahimsa.
2. Satya (Truthfulness): Satya urges us to speak and live our truth. But it's not about brutal honesty. It's about expressing our truth tactfully, in ways that uphold Ahimsa.
3. Asteya (Non-stealing): Asteya goes beyond refraining from theft. It's about not taking what hasn't been freely given, including others' time or ideas, or even imposing our beliefs on them.
4. Brahmacharya (Non-excess): Brahmacharya is about moderating our sensory cravings. It could translate into simple practices like mindful eating, digital detox, or spending time in nature to reconnect with ourselves.
5. Aparigraha (Non-possessiveness): Aparigraha encourages us to let go of our attachments, be it material possessions or our own expectations and biases. Practicing gratitude can be a wonderful way to cultivate this principle.

Niyamas: The Five Personal Observances

1. While Yamas guide us in our social interactions, Niyamas are more personal, guiding our inner spiritual journey.
2. Saucha (Purity): Saucha is about maintaining external and internal purity. This could mean keeping our environment clean, eating healthy, or clearing our mind through meditation.
3. Santosha (Contentment): Santosha is about finding contentment in the present moment, without constantly seeking external validation or possessions.
4. Tapas (Discipline): Tapas is about cultivating self-discipline and resilience. This could be setting a regular yoga or meditation routine, or sticking to a healthy habit.
5. Svadhyaya (Self-study): Svadhyaya encourages us to learn about ourselves, our patterns, and behaviors. This could involve journaling, therapy, or self-reflection.
6. Ishvara Pranidhana (Surrender): This Niyama teaches us to surrender to the divine or a higher power, reminding us that we are a small part of the grand cosmos.

Integrating Yamas and Niyamas into Your Life

How can we make these principles a part of our daily lives? It starts with self-awareness. Reflect on each principle and observe your actions and thoughts. Where could you incorporate more Ahimsa or Santosha? How can you practice Aparigraha in your daily interactions? As you ponder these principles, consider the following questions:

1. Which Yama or Niyama resonates with you the most?
2. Can you identify a situation where you practiced one of these principles?
3. How could you apply these principles more consciously in your life?

Remember, it's not about perfection, but progress. It's okay to stumble

Bringing Yogic Philosophy into Everyday Life: Exercises and Practices

Integrating the principles of yogic philosophy into daily life can feel like navigating a labyrinth. However, with practice, you'll see a beautiful unfolding of personal transformation and cultivation of your inner light. Let's explore some exercises and practices to guide you on this path.

Mindfulness: The Key to Inner Light

Practicing mindfulness is like lighting a candle within yourself. Every time your awareness expands, the light grows brighter, illuminating the hidden corners of your mind. Engaging in mindfulness exercises such as meditation or mindful eating can help ground you in the present moment, creating a strong foundation for your yogic journey.

Journaling: A Mirror to Your Soul

Journaling is an excellent tool for reflecting on your journey and tracking your progress. Consider maintaining a 'Yoga Philosophy Journal' where you jot down your reflections on the Yamas, Niyamas, or any other aspects of yogic philosophy that you're exploring. This personal record can serve as a powerful tool for self-discovery and can help you identify patterns or areas where you need to focus more.

Daily Affirmations: Cultivating Positivity

Daily affirmations are positive statements that can help you change your negative self-talk and nurture a more positive outlook towards life. For instance, you could choose an affirmation based on a Yama or Niyama that resonates with you. Repeat this affirmation daily, especially during moments of silence or meditation.

Physical Yoga: A Moving Meditation

Physical yoga, or asana practice, is a wonderful way to embody yogic philosophy. Whether it's practicing Ahimsa through a nurturing yoga sequence or Aparigraha by letting go of the desire to perfect a pose, asanas can offer a unique way to integrate philosophy into your physical body.

Creating a Conducive Environment

Now that you have an idea of the practices you can engage in, it's crucial to create a space conducive to nurturing these habits. Dedicate a quiet corner of your home for your yoga and mindfulness practices. Keep your journal and a pen handy. Make sure the space is clean and clutter-free, reflecting the principle of Saucha.

Tracking Your Progress

To help you keep track of your journey, consider creating a checklist or a worksheet where you note down your daily practices. This can include your mindfulness exercises, the affirmation you chose for the day, or your reflections from journaling.

Remember, the journey of incorporating yogic philosophy into daily life is a personal and ongoing one. The progress is slow, but every step you take on this path brings you closer to your true self, enhances your inner light, and transforms your life in remarkable ways. So, take a deep breath, be patient with yourself, and embark on this enlightening journey.

The Eight Limbs of Yoga: An Overview

The Eight Limbs of Yoga: A Holistic Path to Inner Light

Yoga is much more than just physical postures; it's a holistic system of well-being that encompasses mind, body, and spirit. This comprehensive system is represented by the Eight Limbs of Yoga, also known as Ashtanga, from the ancient text, the Yoga Sutras of Patanjali. Let's take a journey through each of these limbs, exploring their interconnectedness and their role in nurturing your inner light.

Yama: Social Ethics

The first limb, Yama, concerns social ethics—how we interact with the world. It consists of five principles: Ahimsa (non-violence), Satya (truthfulness), Asteya (non-stealing), Brahmacharya (moderation), and Aparigraha (non-covetousness). Applying these principles encourages us to lead a life of integrity and kindness.

Niyama: Personal Practices

Niyama, the second limb, focuses on personal practices that cultivate self-discipline and inner strength. These are Saucha (purity), Santosha (contentment), Tapas (discipline), Svadhyaya (self-study), and Ishvara Pranidhana (surrender to a higher power).

Asana: Physical Postures

Asana, the third limb and probably the most recognizable, involves the practice of physical postures. It's through asanas that we build strength, flexibility, and balance, facilitating a harmonious connection between mind and body.

Pranayama: Breath Control

The fourth limb, Pranayama, involves controlling the breath. It is through Pranayama that we learn to harness the vital life force (prana), bringing about mental clarity and tranquillity.

Pratyahara: Sensory Withdrawal

Pratyahara, the fifth limb, involves withdrawal from sensory distractions to turn our focus inward. This practice enhances our ability to concentrate and prepares us for meditation.

Dharana: Concentration

Dharana, the sixth limb, is the practice of concentration, where we learn to steady the mind by focusing on a single object, mantra, or thought.

Dhyana: Meditation

The seventh limb, Dhyana, is meditative absorption, where the practitioner becomes fully engaged in the focus of their concentration.

Samadhi: Blissful Union

Samadhi, the eighth and final limb, is a state of blissful union with the divine or one's true self.

Integrating the Eight Limbs into Daily Life

Now that we have explored each limb, it's important to understand that these aren't steps to be mastered in order, but rather they interact and weave together, each supporting and informing the others. Think of them as threads in a tapestry, each equally crucial in creating the complete picture of your yogic journey.

To integrate these principles into your daily life, start small. Choose one Yama and one Niyama to focus on each week. Incorporate a short meditation into your daily routine. Dedicate time to your asana practice, and remember to sync your movements with your breath.

Test Your Understanding

Let's test your understanding of the Eight Limbs with a quick quiz. What are the five Yamas? Can you distinguish between Dharana and Dhyana? Which limb focuses on breath control? Remember, there's no rush. The journey through the Eight Limbs is a lifelong practice, offering endless opportunities for learning and growth.

Meditation: How Different Meditation Techniques Can Be Used to Cultivate Inner Light

Meditation, in its myriad forms, is an essential part of yoga practice, illuminating the pathway to inner light. It helps us go beyond our noisy thoughts and access a state of stillness and clarity. Let's delve deeper into different meditation techniques that can help nurture your inner radiance.

Breathing Meditation: The Power of the Breath

Our journey starts with the simplest yet profound technique, Breathing Meditation. Often overlooked, our breath is a potent tool to navigate the fluctuating currents of our mind. By merely observing your breath—its rhythm, depth, temperature—you are anchoring yourself in the present. This mindful practice serves as a beacon, guiding you towards inner tranquility and light.

Visualization Meditation: Picturing Light Within

Visualization meditation, introduced in Chapter 1, involves creating a mental image to foster positivity. To enhance your inner light, imagine a radiant sun within your heart, glowing brighter with each breath. Envision this light spreading through your body, infusing every cell with warmth, love, and vitality. This powerful technique transforms your inner landscape, sparking joy and serenity.

Mantra Meditation: Sound Vibrations to Illuminate Within

Mantra meditation employs repetitive sounds to quiet the mind and cultivate inner peace. The mantra, a word or phrase, serves as an anchor, helping focus your mind and dispel distraction. Chanting a mantra such as "Om" or "I am light" can attune you to the vibration of inner light, fostering a sense of unity with your true essence.

Body Scan Meditation: Inner Awareness and Light

Body scan meditation, revisited from previous chapters, is a journey of self-awareness. By mindfully scanning your body from head to toe, you acknowledge sensations without judgment. This fosters a loving connection with your body, a vital step towards cultivating inner light.

Complementary Meditations for Your Journey

Observation Meditation: Embracing the Nature Around You

Observation meditation, sometimes known as nature meditation, is a method that encourages mindfulness by paying attention to our surroundings. This practice can bring forth a sense of unity and harmony, ultimately illuminating your inner light.

For this meditation, you'll need to find a quiet spot in nature where you feel comfortable and at ease - it could be your garden, a park, or even a serene corner at your home with a few plants around.

- Here's how to practice Observation Meditation:
  Observe Mindfully: As you engage your senses, stay present. If your mind starts to wander, gently bring it back to the observation.

- Inner Reflection: After a while, close your eyes and reflect inward. How do you feel? Is there a sense of calm and interconnectedness? Can you feel your inner light reflecting the tranquility of nature?

- Closing: Sit quietly for a few moments, acknowledging the peace within you. Slowly open your eyes, bring your hands to your heart, and express gratitude for this moment of connection with nature.

Observation Meditation offers a break from our technologically-driven lives and brings us back to our roots. By mindfully observing nature, we not only enhance our awareness but also stir our inherent connection with the universe, shining our inner light brighter. It's a gentle reminder that we're part of a magnificent larger whole.

Walking Meditation

Introduced in Chapter 2, Walking Meditation is a mindful practice that cultivates presence. Each step taken with awareness strengthens your connection to the world around you, fostering inner light.

Practical Tip: Your Meditation Space

Create a calming meditation environment at home. Dedicate a quiet space, use soft lighting, and perhaps add a few inspiring elements like a plant, a candle, or a motivational quote. This physical space can mirror and support the inner peace and light you're cultivating.

Remember, meditation is a practice. It's less about perfection and more about showing up consistently, creating space to shine your inner light. Let these techniques be your companions as you journey towards your radiant self. Happy meditating!

Guided Journaling Exercise: Reflecting on Meditation Experience

Exploring the Depths of Your Practice

Meditation, as we've discovered in earlier chapters, is a voyage into the unseen terrains of our inner selves. We unearth layers of consciousness, explore the contours of our minds, and embrace our innate luminosity. Journaling these experiences provides us with a map to navigate our inner landscapes, serving as a lighthouse in our spiritual journey.

Harnessing the Power of Observation

During your meditation, what sensations swept through your body? Was there warmth blooming from your core, a vibration pulsating in your fingertips, or perhaps a tingle of energy along your spine? Here's an opportunity to not just observe these sensations but document them. Record your physical experiences post meditation, noting any distinct sensations or lack thereof.

Consider these questions:

1. How did your body feel during and after the practice?
2. What physical sensations can you recall?
3. Did you feel any resistance or ease in certain parts of your body?

Reflecting on these questions not only deepens your self-awareness but also helps tailor your practice, facilitating a more harmonious mind-body connection.

The Inner Light Journal: Recognizing Your Patterns

In the quiet corners of our minds, we often encounter thoughts or emotions that we otherwise overlook. Meditation brings these to the surface, allowing us to engage with them. Documenting these insights helps identify patterns and recurring themes.

Ask yourself:

1. What thoughts kept surfacing during your practice?
2. Were you able to acknowledge and let go of these thoughts, or did you find yourself entwined with them?
3. What emotions arose during and post your meditation session?

Answering these questions will help you recognize patterns, unveiling the brilliance of your inner light.

Practical Tips for Maintaining a Journaling Habit

- **Consistency Is Key**

  The secret to effective journaling lies in its regularity. It need not be a lengthy discourse; just a few reflective lines each day can work wonders. Choose a fixed time, ideally soon after your meditation practice, to ensure that the experiences are fresh in your mind.

- **Embrace the Journey**
  Remember, there's no "perfect" way to journal. Your entries may evolve with time, just as you do. Avoid self-judgment or criticism, for this journey of self-reflection and exploration is as unique as you are.
- **Your Sacred Space**
  Maintain a dedicated journal for your meditation reflections. This not only keeps your thoughts organized but also turns your journal into a sacred space for introspection.

As you step forth on this path of journaling, embrace it as a means of illuminating your journey, making visible the invisible and known the unknown. Use it to navigate through the myriad experiences of meditation, acknowledging the rich tapestry of your consciousness. As you record, reflect, and revisit your experiences, you'll witness the radiance of your inner light growing brighter, guiding you towards self-discovery and, ultimately, self-realization.

The Power of Cultivating Inner Light

As we conclude this chapter, let us delve into the magnificent power of cultivating our inner light. This radiant source within us can be nurtured, stoked, and guided, leading us towards a path of personal growth, self-discovery, and a profound connection to our highest self.

The Luminosity Within: A Beacon of Growth and Discovery

Our inner light, the beacon of our inherent wisdom and authenticity, illuminates our path, both on the yoga mat and in our everyday life. This glow emanates from our core, permeating through our entire being and affecting all aspects of our lives – our decisions, our relationships, our sense of self, and our outlook on the world.

Cultivating this inner light enables us to discern our genuine desires, recognize our strengths, and confront our weaknesses with compassion. It's akin to holding a torch in the labyrinth of self-exploration, lighting the way as we navigate the complex corridors of our psyche.

With consistent practice and commitment to our yoga and meditation journey, we feed this radiant energy, causing it to shine brighter and guide us more effectively. It is our unwavering ally, a lighthouse amidst stormy seas, leading us to our truth and our essence.

Igniting Transformation: A Commitment to Inner Radiance

Embracing the journey of inner light cultivation is akin to planting a seed within your soul. It requires nurturing, patience, and steadfast commitment. The journey may not always be easy, but the transformation it ignites is deeply rewarding.

By aligning with our inner light, we become more resilient, adaptable, and attuned to our inner wisdom. We learn to navigate life's ebbs and flows with grace and acceptance, recognizing that each experience is an opportunity for growth.

With your continued commitment to yoga and meditation, the inner light begins to spill over, infusing your life with a sense of peace, joy, and purpose. And in this radiant glow, you can truly flourish.

Commitment Pledge

As we embark on this lifelong journey, I invite you to make a commitment. A commitment to your practice, to your self-discovery, and to the radiant light within you. Consider this as an action plan, a solemn pledge to nurturing your luminescence.

Grab your journal, find a quiet space, and reflect on these prompts:

1. **Why do I wish to cultivate my inner light?** Recognize your motivation. It could be for self-growth, for better understanding of self, or for a deeper spiritual connection. Write down your "why."
2. **How will I commit to my yoga practice?** Will you dedicate a specific time each day? Maybe you'll explore different yoga styles or meditations to keep your practice vibrant and aligned with your needs. Detail your plan.
3. **What will I do when challenges arise?** There will be days when practice feels heavy, when self-doubt creeps in, or when life throws you off course. How will you navigate these times? Craft your strategy.

Once you've written your answers, formulate your pledge. It could be something like this:

> *"I, [Your Name], commit to cultivating my inner light for [your "why"].*
> *I pledge to honor my yoga and meditation practice by [your plan]. In*
> *times of challenge, I promise to [your strategy], remembering that each*
> *step, no matter how small, is progress on my journey."*

The act of writing this commitment pledge can have a profound effect on your dedication to nurturing your inner light. It provides you with a tangible reminder of your promise to yourself, reaffirming your dedication to this journey of self-discovery.

As we conclude, remember, the radiant light within you is a source of unending strength and wisdom. It is the essence of who you are, your unique spark in this vast universe. This light has the potential to guide you towards self-understanding, compassion, and a profound sense of inner peace..

Embracing the Journey

Just as a seed needs consistent care to bloom, so does your inner light. The journey of self-discovery and growth is not a sprint but a marathon. It's an ongoing commitment to introspection, understanding, and patience with oneself.

Embrace this journey. Each yoga pose, every moment of meditation, every journal entry brings you one step closer to your authentic self, to the bright inner light that resides within you. This path of cultivation may be long, and at times challenging, but the fruits of your labor will be immensely rewarding.

Unleashing Your Inner Radiance

When we commit to cultivating our inner light, we embark on a transformative journey that reaches far beyond our yoga mat. We begin to live more authentically, aligning our actions with our inner truths, and letting our unique light shine brightly in the world.

As your inner light shines brighter, it not only enlightens your path but can serve as a beacon for others, encouraging them to embark on their journeys of self-discovery. The brilliance of your inner light has the potential to illuminate the world in unimaginable ways.

Guiding Light: Looking Forward

As we close this chapter, carry with you the knowledge of the power within you. The cultivation of your inner light is a transformative practice, one that has the potential to guide you to deeper self-understanding and fulfillment.

In the chapters to come, we will delve deeper into the philosophical aspects of yoga, exploring profound teachings that will further illuminate your path. Through these insights, we'll continue to nurture the radiant light within, guiding it to shine brighter with each passing day.

Remember your pledge and reiterate it whenever you need motivation or reassurance. This commitment you've made today marks the beginning of a remarkable journey towards illuminating your true self. So let's move forward, honoring our inner light, guiding it to shine brighter, embarking on this journey of self-discovery and growth together.

As the glow of your inner light grows stronger, may you experience increased clarity, peace, and joy in your journey. Trust in its power, let it guide you, and watch as your world transforms before your very eyes. Here's to illuminating your path and your life with the brilliant radiance of your inner light!

9

Yoga Philosophy for Cultivating Inner Light (Part 2)

Welcome to Chapter 9, where we continue our exploration into the profound philosophy of yoga and its relevance in cultivating our inner light. Building on the foundation laid in the previous chapter, we'll delve deeper into various practices that guide us on our journey to enlightenment.

This chapter is your roadmap to developing a personalized yoga practice that nurtures your inner light. We'll venture beyond the yoga mat, discussing how meditation can be integrated into your everyday life and how self-inquiry can reveal the nature of the Self, thereby leading to a luminous inner glow.

We'll also examine the different paths of yoga - Karma Yoga, Bhakti Yoga, Jnana Yoga, Raja Yoga, and Tantric Yoga - detailing their distinct practices and how they can all guide us toward a radiant inner light. To support this journey, we'll introduce Ayurveda, yoga's sister science, and discuss how its principles can nurture our inner light. Lastly, we'll venture into the realm of energy centers or chakras, learning how they influence our inner light and how we can balance and energize them.

Self-Assessment Quiz

Before we proceed, take a moment to assess your current understanding of yoga practices and their potential for nurturing your inner light. Answer the following questions honestly, using a scale of 1 (least) to 5 (most):

1. How familiar are you with the different paths of yoga (Karma, Bhakti, Jnana, Raja, and Tantric Yoga)?
2. How comfortable are you with integrating meditation into your daily routine?
3. To what extent do you engage in self-inquiry as a part of your spiritual growth?
4. Are you aware of the principles of Ayurveda and how they can support your yoga practice?
5. Do you understand the concept of chakras and their significance in cultivating inner light?

Total your score: _____

This quiz is meant to serve as a benchmark, a snapshot of your understanding before we delve deeper into these topics. As we journey together through this chapter, you'll have the opportunity to expand your knowledge and apply these transformative practices to your own life. Remember, every step taken on this path, no matter how small, brings us closer to the radiant inner light within.

Prepare for a transformative journey as we navigate these intricate philosophies and practices, paving the path for your inner light to shine brighter with each passing day. Let's embark on this journey together, illuminating our lives with the profound wisdom of yoga.

Incorporating Meditation into Everyday Life -

Meditation, a pillar of yoga philosophy, is more than an isolated practice reserved for a specific time or place. Its power can seep into the crevices of our everyday lives, serving as a calming beacon amidst the chaos. Here, we'll explore practical ways of integrating meditation into your daily routine, turning ordinary moments into opportunities for mindfulness.

Carving Out Time

The first step in integrating meditation into everyday life is setting aside time for it. It might seem challenging, given our hectic schedules, but remember, you don't need to allocate hours. Even a few minutes of mindful focus can yield profound benefits.

Try to begin or end your day with meditation, creating a tranquil buffer between your inner world and external responsibilities. Morning meditation can set a peaceful tone for the day, while an evening session can help you unwind, processing the day's events with calm introspection.

Infusing Mindfulness into Daily Activities

Beyond dedicated meditation sessions, you can also bring mindfulness to everyday tasks. This practice, often called 'informal meditation,' allows you to convert mundane moments into mindful ones. Whether you're washing dishes, walking the dog, or even brushing your teeth, you can approach these activities with a meditative mindset, focusing on your breath, movements, and sensations. This approach transforms simple tasks into moments of calm and clarity, and your daily routine into an ongoing meditation.

Overcoming Obstacles: Practical Tips

The path to consistent meditation practice isn't without its challenges. Let's explore some common obstacles and tips to overcome them.

1. Time Constraint: If finding a chunk of uninterrupted time feels impossible, try 'micro-meditations.' These are short bursts of mindfulness, maybe just a minute or two, sprinkled throughout your day.
2. Distractions: In our hyper-connected world, distractions are inevitable. Consider them not as disruptions, but as part of your practice. When you notice your attention wavering, gently guide it back without judgment. With time, you'll cultivate a more focused, resilient mind.
3. Expectations: Meditation isn't about achieving a 'blank mind' or immediate peace. It's about observing your thoughts and feelings without getting caught up in them. Let go of expectations and embrace the journey, moment by moment.

Reflection Time:

To better understand how you can incorporate meditation into your life, reflect on the following questions:

1. What time of day would be the most feasible for you to practice meditation? How can you adjust your schedule to accommodate this?
2. What daily activities can you transform into moments of mindfulness?
3. What challenges do you anticipate in maintaining a regular meditation practice? How might you apply the tips above to overcome these?

Remember to jot down your responses in your journal. Reflecting on these questions and documenting your answers will help you create a tailored strategy to integrate meditation into your daily life, nurturing your inner light with every mindful moment. In the end, the path to cultivating inner light is not about grand gestures or radical changes, but about embracing mindfulness in each moment, allowing meditation to softly illuminate our everyday lives.

Self-Inquiry: Exploring the Nature of the Self and How It Can Lead to Cultivating Inner Light

At the heart of yoga philosophy lies a profound practice: Self-Inquiry, a contemplative exploration into the depths of our own existence. By understanding our true nature, we uncover the inner light that yoga encourages us to cultivate. Let's delve into this transformative process.

What is Self-Inquiry?

Self-Inquiry, known as 'Atma Vichara' in Sanskrit, is a philosophical tool for discerning the reality of our true self. It involves peeling back the layers of our identity - our thoughts, emotions, and physicality - to reveal the unchanging essence beneath: the Self.

While our transient identities shift like shadows, the Self remains steady, like the flame of a lamp in a windless place. Recognizing this enduring flame within us is the goal of Self-Inquiry. It illuminates our path, guiding us towards peace, clarity, and unity with the universal consciousness.

Initiate the Process: Practical Steps

Self-Inquiry might sound daunting, but the process is surprisingly straightforward. It starts with an introspective question, often phrased as, "Who am I?"

Step 1: Take some quiet time for yourself, sitting comfortably in a peaceful space. Close your eyes and take a few deep, grounding breaths.

Step 2: Gently ask yourself, "Who am I?" Let the question resonate within you.

Step 3: As thoughts, emotions, and identifications surface, observe them without judgment or engagement. Each time, return to your fundamental question: "Who am I?"

Step 4: Over time, the clamor of temporary identifications quietens, revealing the constant flame of your true Self.

Self-Inquiry is not a one-time practice. It's a lifelong journey that deepens over time, illuminating your path towards inner peace and fulfillment. Remember, the aim is not to analyze or intellectualize, but to simply observe and witness.

Journal for Self-Inquiry

As you embark on this journey of Self-Inquiry, journaling can be an insightful ally. Here are some prompts to facilitate your exploration, distinct from those we've used in previous chapters:

1. When you ask yourself "Who am I?", what initial thoughts and feelings arise? Write them down.
2. How do these self-identifications shift during different moments of your day or various circumstances?
3. As you peel back these layers of identity, what do you start to perceive beneath them?
4. What challenges do you encounter during Self-Inquiry? How can you navigate these in future sessions?
5. How does your perception of yourself shift as you engage with Self-Inquiry over time?

Recording your observations, thoughts, and feelings in response to these prompts will assist you in discerning patterns and deepening your understanding of your Self.

Unleashing Inner Light through Self-Inquiry

By investigating our true nature through Self-Inquiry, we light up the lamp of self-awareness, illuminating our life's path. As we identify less with our transient selves and more with our unchanging essence, we find a peace that transcends everyday worries and woes. We become more resilient, more compassionate, and more unified — both within ourselves and with the world around us.

The journey of Self-Inquiry, like that of yoga, is one of returning home to our true nature. It is a journey into the heart of our being, where we encounter the brilliant light that shines within us. And in this light, we find our truth, our peace, and our unity with the cosmos. It is this inner light that yoga encourages us to cultivate, guiding us towards a life of clarity, peace, and purpose.

Exploring Different Yoga Practices and Their Role in Cultivating Inner Light

The radiant landscape of yoga philosophy is marked by various paths that lead towards a singular, luminous destination: inner light. While the terrain may differ, each path nurtures self-awareness and spiritual growth, cultivating an inner brilliance that guides our journey.

Imagine each path as a different color, illuminating the prism of yoga in its own unique hue. Karma Yoga, the path of selfless service, radiates a golden light, infusing our actions with purpose and compassion. Bhakti Yoga, the path of devotion, glows a passionate red, kindling the flame of love in our hearts.

Then there's Jnana Yoga, the path of wisdom, beaming a clear, bright white - it seeks to dissolve ignorance and illuminate our understanding of reality. Raja Yoga, the path of mental and physical control, shines a calm blue, guiding us towards inner peace and equanimity.

Finally, Tantric Yoga, the path of embracing all aspects of life, emanates a vibrant, inclusive rainbow, reminding us that the sacred interweaves every aspect of our existence.

Each of these practices offers unique ways to cultivate our inner light, enriching our yoga journey. As we venture along these paths, we are not confined to a single route; instead, we find the hues of our yoga practice shifting and blending, much like the changing colors of a sunrise. And it is in this radiant dawn, we find ourselves gradually awakened to the resplendent light within.

Karma Yoga: The Practice of Selfless Service

What is Karma Yoga?

Karma Yoga, often referred to as the 'yoga of action,' is a spiritual practice that focuses on selfless service. Rooted in the word 'Karma', which translates to 'action,' this branch of yoga is about performing deeds without attachment to their outcomes. It's about letting your actions be guided by love and goodwill, rather than ego or expectation of reward.

Think of a candle lighting another. The original candle's light doesn't diminish; instead, it spreads light to another area. This symbolizes the essence of Karma Yoga: by selflessly serving others, we don't lose anything. On the contrary, we enhance our own inner light, as we help others illuminate theirs.

The Role of Karma Yoga in Cultivating Inner Light

In the realm of Karma Yoga, our actions become a form of meditation, a spiritual practice illuminating our understanding of the interconnectedness of all beings. Through selfless service, we tap into the inherent compassion within us, peeling away the layers of ego and revealing our true self – the source of our inner light.

Practical Implementation of Karma Yoga

The practice of Karma Yoga doesn't necessarily mean you have to engage in grand gestures of philanthropy. It can be as simple as helping a neighbor with their groceries, volunteering at a local charity, or showing kindness to a stranger. The key is to act with a genuine sense of selflessness, with no expectation of recognition or reward.

To integrate Karma Yoga into your daily life:

- **Identify Opportunities:** Look for opportunities to help in your immediate environment. Small acts of kindness can have a big impact.

- **Detach from Outcomes:** Perform your actions without attachment to the result. The reward is in the act itself, not the outcome.

- **Act with Love and Goodwill:** Let every action be guided by goodwill and love, rather than ego or expectation of reward.

Interactive Quiz: Test Your Understanding of Karma Yoga

1. How does the philosophy of Karma Yoga interpret the act of giving?

    a) A depletion of one's own resources.

    b) A trade for future benefits.

    c) A neutral action.

    d) A way of enhancing one's own inner light.

2. Why is detachment from the outcome crucial in Karma Yoga?

    a) It allows the focus to remain on the act itself, not the result.

    b) It prevents disappointment.

    c) It encourages an indifferent attitude.

    d) None of the above.

By exploring Karma Yoga, you're not only helping others, but also shining a light within, illuminating your path towards greater self-understanding and compassion. This practice, while simple in concept, can profoundly impact your yoga journey, leading you closer to the radiant inner light of your true self.

Bhakti Yoga: The Practice of Devotion

Understanding Bhakti Yoga

Bhakti Yoga, often termed as the 'yoga of devotion,' is an emotional, spiritual path where love and devotion towards a higher power are the guiding principles. While the object of this devotion may vary, the essence remains the same: unconditional love, pure devotion, and surrender. Picture a river flowing into the sea, losing itself in the process, yet becoming part of something vast and infinite. That's the transformative journey of a Bhakti yogi.

Cultivating Inner Light Through Bhakti Yoga

Bhakti Yoga has a profound role in igniting the inner light. As you embark on this practice, your heart opens to unconditional love and devotion, casting away the shadows of ego, judgment, and fear. Like a lamp glowing in the darkness, your inner light brightens, guided by love and surrender. This spiritual love is powerful; it illuminates your being, bringing forth compassion, kindness, and inner peace.

Incorporating Bhakti Yoga into Your Practice

Practicing Bhakti Yoga can be a deeply personal journey, here are some ways to infuse it into your daily life:

Chanting and Singing: Songs of devotion, also known as 'Bhajans' or 'Kirtan,' can help evoke feelings of love and adoration.

Prayer and Meditation: Regularly spending time in prayer or meditation can help cultivate a deep sense of devotion.

Seva (Service): Unconditional service to others, without expecting anything in return, is a powerful way of practicing Bhakti Yoga.

Study of Sacred Texts: Reading spiritual texts can provide deeper insight into the nature of devotion and guide your practice.

Quiz: Your Understanding of Bhakti Yoga

1. What metaphor best represents the journey of a Bhakti Yogi?

    a) A tree growing towards the sunlight.

    b) A river flowing into the sea.

    c) A bird flying in the sky.

    d) A mountain standing tall.

2. How does Bhakti Yoga contribute to the cultivation of inner light?

    a) Through physical strength and flexibility.

    b) Through intellectual knowledge and wisdom.

    c) Through the practice of devotion and unconditional love.

    d) Through daily chores and responsibilities.

By immersing yourself in Bhakti Yoga, the practice of devotion, you allow your heart to expand in the vast ocean of spiritual love. As your inner light brightens, fueled by this unconditional love, you may find a transformative sense of peace and fulfillment that permeates every aspect of your life.

Jnana Yoga: The Practice of Wisdom

Grasping Jnana Yoga

Jnana Yoga, the yoga of wisdom or knowledge, is the journey towards self-realization through discernment and understanding. It is not just knowledge in the traditional sense, but profound inner wisdom that dispels the illusion of separateness and connects us with the universal truth of oneness.

Lighting the Inner Lamp with Jnana Yoga

When we talk about the inner light, Jnana Yoga becomes a powerful torch illuminating the path. Through introspection and self-inquiry, you're peeling away layers of misconception, bias, and illusion. The clearer your vision becomes, the brighter your inner light shines. Jnana Yoga is not just about gaining knowledge, but about using that knowledge to discern the real from the unreal, the eternal from the temporary.

Practical Steps to Implement Jnana Yoga

Implementing Jnana Yoga involves a combination of study, reflection, and meditation:

Study of Sacred Texts: Dive into spiritual texts like the Upanishads or Bhagavad Gita. Let these profound words guide your journey towards wisdom.

Self-inquiry: Consistently ask questions like "Who am I?" or "What is my true nature?" This self-inquiry (Atma Vichara) can be an eye-opening experience.

Meditation: Regular meditation helps clear the mind and allows for deeper reflection and understanding.

Test Your Understanding: Jnana Yoga Quiz

1. What does Jnana Yoga primarily focus on achieving?

    a) Physical wellness.

    b) A sense of service and duty.

    c) A clear understanding of reality.

d) Financial prosperity.

2. What forms the core of self-inquiry in Jnana Yoga?

    a) Asking questions about worldly affairs.

    b) Questioning one's identity and true nature.

    c) Analyzing others' behaviors.

    d) None of the above.

In embracing Jnana Yoga, you're embarking on a journey towards self-realization through wisdom. It's a challenging path, demanding deep introspection and analysis. However, the rewards are transformative, as it enables you to see the world in its true form, and in this understanding, your inner light shines brighter than ever before.

Raja Yoga: The Practice of Mental and Physical Control

The Royal Path: Understanding Raja Yoga

Raja Yoga, often termed as the "Royal Path," represents the practice of mental and physical control. It's a holistic journey that encapsulates all the other forms of yoga, focusing on controlling the mind and body to cultivate the inner light.

Harnessing Inner Light with Raja Yoga

Imagine a serene lake, its surface untouched by ripples. This tranquility is what Raja Yoga seeks to bring to our minds. By taming the churning thoughts and emotions, it brings clarity, letting our inner light shine brightly. It's the pursuit of self-mastery - an ultimate union of the individual self with the universal self.

Practical Steps to Implement Raja Yoga

Raja Yoga follows the Eight Limbs of Yoga outlined by Patanjali in the Yoga Sutras:

> **Yama and Niyama:** These ethical principles guide our actions and behaviors.
>
> **Asana:** Regular physical postures help control the body and mind.
>
> **Pranayama:** Control of breath aids in balancing energy.
>
> **Pratyahara:** Withdrawal of senses allows for internal focus.

Dharana: Concentration paves the way for deep meditation.

Dhyana: Deep meditation leads to a state of peace.

Samadhi: The final stage of deep contemplation and unity with the universal self.

Quiz Time: Raja Yoga

1. Raja Yoga is often referred to as the "Royal Path." Why?

    a) It was originally practiced by royalty.

    b) It's more complex than other forms of yoga.

    c) It encompasses all other forms of yoga.

    d) None of the above.

2. How does Raja Yoga affect the practitioner's state of mind?

    a) It creates a constant state of excitement and anticipation.

    b) It brings tranquility and control over emotions and thoughts.

    c) It encourages a state of constant worry and awareness.

    d) None of the above.

Raja Yoga is a holistic approach, encompassing ethical living, physical wellbeing, and mental clarity. When practised consistently, this royal path leads us to a state of serene introspection, where our inner light can shine unobstructed. It's a journey of personal discipline and mastery, an invitation to truly know and connect with ourselves. Remember, the journey is the destination. Every step taken in mindfulness brings us closer to our radiant inner light.

Tantric Yoga: The Practice of Embracing All Aspects of Life

A Deeper Look into Tantric Yoga

In the varied tapestry of yoga traditions, Tantric Yoga shines as a rich and empowering practice. Unlike some other styles that may focus on renunciation, Tantric Yoga encourages the full embrace of life in all its aspects. It intertwines the physical, mental, and spiritual, suggesting that our everyday experiences can be stepping stones towards higher consciousness.

How It Works

Tantric Yoga proposes that everything in our existence – from the grandeur of nature's landscapes to the routine of our daily tasks – contains a spark of the divine. By learning to see and celebrate this sacred essence, we enrich our lives and hasten our spiritual progress. This practice is not about mastering complex postures but rather cultivating a unique state of awareness.

Practical Steps for Implementation

Mindfulness in Daily Activities: Start to view ordinary tasks as sacred rituals. Whether you're washing dishes, commuting, or eating, do it with complete presence and reverence.

Meditation and Visualization: Regularly spend time in silence and introspection. Visualize the energy channels in your body, awakening and harmonizing them.

Physical Practice: Tantric Yoga also involves specific postures (asanas) and breathwork (pranayama). Engage in these practices under the guidance of an experienced teacher to ensure safe and effective practice.

Your Turn: Engage with the Practice

Ready to try? Start by bringing mindfulness into a simple daily task. For one week, choose one activity each day, and commit to performing it with full awareness. Note any changes in your attitude or feelings afterward.

Quiz Yourself

1. How does Tantric Yoga view ordinary daily tasks?

    a) As mundane activities to be completed quickly.

    b) As distractions from spiritual growth.

    c) As sacred rituals that can enhance spiritual awareness.

    d) As tasks best delegated to others.

2. What is the purpose of visualization in Tantric Yoga?

   a) To enhance creativity and imagination.

   b) To awaken and harmonize energy channels in the body.

   c) To plan for future events and circumstances.

   d) None of the above.

Remember, Tantric Yoga is about inclusivity, experiencing the sacred in the mundane, and celebrating life fully. As you engage with this practice, you are invited to appreciate your journey's unique and diverse aspects, igniting your inner light.

Ayurveda: The Sister Science of Yoga and How It Can Be Used to Support the Cultivation of Inner Light

Introduction to Ayurveda and its Relationship with Yoga

Just as the moon shares an unbreakable bond with the night sky, Ayurveda is inseparably linked to Yoga. Born from the same philosophical roots in ancient India, they are often referred to as sister sciences. While Yoga directs its energy towards spiritual elevation, Ayurveda focuses on health and well-being, forming a holistic approach to living. They both share the ultimate goal of achieving harmony, illuminating the inner light within us.

Ayurveda, translating to 'the science of life,' understands the world as an interplay of energies. It teaches that our health and well-being depend on a delicate balance between the mind, body, and spirit. Each person is seen as a unique blend of the three fundamental bio-energies, or 'doshas': Vata (air and space), Pitta (fire and water), and Kapha (earth and water). Understanding and honoring our unique constitution can guide us towards a more harmonious, vibrant life.

Practical Tips: Incorporating Ayurvedic Principles into Daily Life

Understand Your Unique Constitution: Identifying your dominant dosha can illuminate your strengths, susceptibilities, and the types of practices and lifestyle choices that are most supportive for you.

Harmonize with Nature's Rhythms: Ayurveda teaches us to align our activities with the rhythms of nature – rising with the sun, eating our main meal when the sun is highest, and winding down as the sun sets.

Cultivate a Balanced Diet: Ayurveda recommends a balanced diet according to one's dosha. For example, a Pitta-dominant individual might favor cool, dry, and sweet foods to counterbalance their inherent fire.

Practice Mindful Living: Just as Yoga promotes mindful movements, Ayurveda encourages mindfulness in our daily activities, urging us to eat, work, and rest with full awareness and presence.

Integrate Ayurvedic Self-care Rituals: These might include self-massage, oil pulling, tongue scraping, and nasal irrigation.

Discover Your Dosha

To gain insights into your Ayurvedic constitution, consider the following self-assessment. While it won't provide a definitive diagnosis, it can guide you towards a deeper understanding of your inherent nature.

Physical Structure: Are you naturally slender and find it hard to gain weight (Vata), have a medium, muscular build (Pitta), or have a larger frame and gain weight easily (Kapha)?

Personality Traits: Are you lively and enthusiastic, but also tend to be anxious (Vata), confident and passionate, but sometimes intense or irritable (Pitta), or calm and caring, but prone to procrastination (Kapha)?

Response to Stress: Do you tend to become anxious and worry (Vata), become angry or frustrated (Pitta), or withdraw and avoid confrontation (Kapha)?

Add up your responses for each dosha. The dosha with the most points is likely your dominant dosha. Remember, this is a simplified assessment, and a professional Ayurvedic practitioner can provide a comprehensive evaluation.

In conclusion, by embracing Ayurvedic principles, we can nurture our physical well-being, which, in turn, supports our Yogic journey. This holistic approach invites us to live mindfully and in harmony with our inherent nature, illuminating our path towards the cultivation of inner light.

Understanding and Working with Energy Centers (Chakras) for Cultivating Inner Light

An Introduction to the Concept of Chakras and Their Significance in Cultivating Inner Light

Like a rainbow in the sky, the body is adorned with seven energy centers, known as Chakras. Rooted in ancient yogic traditions, the Chakras are believed to be whirlpools of energy where our physical and spiritual selves intersect. Each Chakra resonates with a different aspect of our being and, when balanced, they contribute to a harmonious sense of well-being, aiding in the cultivation of inner light.

Starting from the base of the spine and ascending to the crown of the head, the seven Chakras are:

1. **Muladhara (Root Chakra):** Instills feelings of safety and grounding.
2. **Svadhisthana (Sacral Chakra):** Governs creativity and emotional balance.
3. **Manipura (Solar Plexus Chakra):** Embodies personal power and confidence.
4. **Anahata (Heart Chakra):** Fosters love and compassion.
5. **Vishuddha (Throat Chakra):** Encourages authentic communication.
6. **Ajna (Third Eye Chakra):** Enhances intuition and insight.
7. **Sahasrara (Crown Chakra):** Connects us to our higher consciousness and spirituality.

Practical Tip: Techniques for Balancing and Energizing Each Chakra

- **Yoga Poses:** Specific yoga poses can be used to activate and balance each Chakra. For instance, Tree Pose (Vrikshasana) for the Root Chakra, or Shoulder Stand (Sarvangasana) for the Throat Chakra.

- **Meditation:** Visualizing the color associated with each Chakra (starting with red for the Root Chakra and moving up to violet for the Crown Chakra) can help in balancing them.
- **Mantras & Chants:** Chanting specific sounds or mantras can stimulate each Chakra. For example, 'LAM' for the Root Chakra and 'HAM' for the Throat Chakra.
- **Diet:** Eating foods that correspond to each Chakra's color can also aid in balancing. Root vegetables for the Root Chakra, for instance, or blueberries for the Third Eye Chakra.

A Guided Visualization Exercise for Working with Chakras

Now, let's embark on a brief journey through our Chakras. Find a quiet, comfortable space where you can relax and close your eyes.

1. Start by visualizing a warm, red glow at the base of your spine, your Root Chakra. Feel it grounding you, connecting you to the earth.
2. Let this light rise, turning into an orange glow at your Sacral Chakra. Feel it spark creativity and emotional balance.
3. Continue to the Solar Plexus Chakra, picturing a yellow light. Allow it to fill you with confidence and personal power.
4. Let this energy rise to your heart, where it transforms into a green glow. Allow feelings of love and compassion to fill your being.
5. As the energy moves to your throat, see a blue light. Feel it encouraging clear, authentic communication.
6. Move this energy to your Third Eye Chakra, visualizing an indigo light. Let it enhance your intuition and insight.
7. Finally, let the energy rise to the top of your head, your Crown Chakra. Here, it becomes a violet light, connecting you to your higher consciousness.

By cultivating an understanding and practice around our Chakras, we can align ourselves with our intrinsic nature and enhance the inner light within us.

Take a few moments in each visualization to really feel the energy and the unique attributes each chakra brings to your overall well-being.

When you've completed your journey from the Root Chakra to the Crown Chakra, spend a few moments in silence, integrating the energy and sensations you've cultivated during the practice. You may feel a renewed sense of balance and alignment in your physical and emotional states, a subtle inner light glowing brighter from within.

Remember, this is your journey, unique to you. There is no right or wrong way to experience your chakras. Some days, certain chakras might feel more active or stagnant, and that's perfectly okay. The goal is not perfection, but increased awareness and attunement to your own energetic body.

This guided visualization can be done as often as you like. It can serve as a powerful tool to start your day or as a soothing practice to end your day, helping to realign your chakras and cultivate your inner light.

Working with our chakras can serve as a powerful complement to our yoga practice, enabling us to balance our energies, enhance our mental and physical well-being, and most importantly, cultivate our inner light. Understanding these energy centers and learning how to balance them will bring us one step closer to achieving unity between our body, mind, and spirit, the ultimate goal of yoga.

In the pursuit of inner light, remember, yoga and its related practices aren't just exercises or tasks to be completed. They're part of a journey, a transformative process of self-discovery and self-improvement. The path may not always be easy, but the rewards—enhanced self-awareness, inner peace, and a deeper connection to the world around us—are worth the effort.

The Power of Cultivating Inner Light through Yoga

Throughout this chapter, we've embarked on a journey of discovery, exploring complex aspects of Yoga and its sister science, Ayurveda. We've shed light on the Chakras, learned to balance our unique constitutions, and cultivated our inner light. It's now time to reflect on this transformative power that Yoga holds, guiding us towards self-discovery and fostering an inherent sense of peace and harmony.

Reflection: Yoga's Transformative Journey

Just like how the Yoga mat serves as a microcosm for life's lessons, every practice, every breath, and every pose you engage with are steps towards your self-transformation. Each asana is a mirror, reflecting back to us our strengths, our challenges, and our infinite potential. As you've moved through the practices in this chapter, you may have noticed shifts within yourself, a subtle glow emanating from within, an inner light growing brighter.

Encouragement: Sustaining the Practice

Remember, cultivating inner light is a continuous journey. The practices of Yoga and Ayurveda are not finite tasks to be completed, but ongoing practices to be explored and integrated into your life. I encourage you to continue on this path, to learn, to grow, and to shine. Let these practices be the beacon that guides you through life's ups and downs, lighting the path towards greater self-awareness and peace.

Your Yoga Action Plan

As we conclude this chapter, it's time for you to take the reins. Consider how you can incorporate the practices discussed in this chapter into your daily life. Use the following template to create your personalized Yoga Action Plan:

1. What practices resonated with you the most in this chapter?
2. How can you integrate these practices into your daily routine?
3. What obstacles might come up, and how can you address them?
4. How will you track your progress and make necessary adjustments?

Reflect on these questions and fill out your action plan. Keep it somewhere you can regularly see and revisit it. Adjust it as necessary, and remember to be gentle with yourself as you embark on this journey.

As we transition into the next chapter, we bring with us the illuminating power of yoga, the practice that not only fosters physical wellness but mental clarity and emotional balance. We carry with us our inner light, nurtured and cultivated through our practices. Our journey isn't over yet. It's time now to move deeper, to explore the nexus of Yoga and inner wisdom, to uncover the intuitive, spiritual aspects of our beings. We'll delve into the process of unearthing this wisdom, acknowledging that the path may not be straightforward but is nonetheless integral to personal growth and self-discovery. Remember, the light of Yoga shines brightly, always guiding you towards the path of inner wisdom. Let's embark on this journey together in the next chapter.

10

Honoring Your Inner Wisdom

As we stand at the threshold of this new chapter, we take with us the empowering knowledge of yoga and its transformative effects, lighting the way from within. The practices we've explored have opened doors, not only to physical wellness but mental clarity and emotional balance. Now, with that inner light shining brightly, it's time to harness that energy and direct it towards a deeper understanding of our own intuition, our inner wisdom.

The Nexus of Yoga and Inner Wisdom

Yoga isn't just about the physical. It's about the spiritual, the mental, the emotional, and the intuitive. It's about cultivating an awareness of your true self - your inner wisdom. The journey to uncover this wisdom isn't always straightforward, but it's an integral part of personal growth and self-discovery. And that's what we'll explore in this chapter.

The Power of Inner Wisdom

Within you resides a unique and intuitive voice, one that carries the whispers of your authentic self. This is your inner wisdom - a guiding force that nudges you in the right direction when you're lost, a beacon that shines through the fog of uncertainty. Learning to listen and honor this voice is a journey that yoga can facilitate, weaving together the threads of mindfulness, acceptance, and deep self-awareness.

Unearthing Your Inner Wisdom

Before we can honor our inner wisdom, we must first recognize and understand it. Yoga, with its emphasis on deep introspection and presence, provides the ideal environment for this exploration. As we peel back the layers of our consciousness through meditation and asanas, we begin to unearth the wisdom buried within.

Inner Wisdom Self-Assessment

To better understand where you stand in your journey of discovering and honoring your inner wisdom, let's take a moment for reflection. This self-assessment quiz will help you gauge your current understanding of your inner wisdom, its voice in your life, and how yoga can help amplify it.

Remember, this journey is yours alone, so take it at your own pace. Whether you're at the beginning or well into your adventure, every step brings you closer to knowing and honoring your true self, your inner wisdom. Let yoga be the compass that guides you on this rewarding path.

Understanding the Concept of Inner Wisdom

What is Inner Wisdom?

Inner wisdom is our intuitive understanding, a form of inborn guidance system. It's an inherent knowledge that extends beyond the conscious mind and rational thinking, connecting us to our authentic selves. When we tap into this source, we align with our true desires, needs, and potential, leading to more fulfilling and balanced lives.

Inner Wisdom in Our Lives

Our inner wisdom acts as a compass, guiding us through life's complexities. It's our gut feeling when we meet a stranger, the quiet voice urging us to take a break when we're overworked, or the deep-seated conviction telling us to pursue a dream against all odds. By connecting with and trusting our inner wisdom, we can make decisions more confidently and lead more authentic, fulfilling lives.

Discovering My Inner Wisdom

Let me share a story about my dear friend, David. David was a dedicated lawyer, always striving for the best. However, he often felt overwhelmed and unsatisfied, despite his professional success. In search of solace, he ventured into the world of yoga and meditation.

One day, during a deep meditation, he had an epiphany. He realized that his true passion was not law, but teaching. His love for sharing knowledge and guiding others was his inner wisdom pointing towards his true path. Trusting his intuition, he decided to take a leap of faith and transitioned into an educational career.

Today, David is a happier, more fulfilled individual. As an educator, he's impacting lives and finding immense satisfaction in his work. His story exemplifies how listening to our inner wisdom can lead to profound, positive changes in our lives.

Tapping into Your Inner Wisdom

The journey to understanding and trusting our inner wisdom is deeply personal and unique. It involves self-reflection, mindfulness, and the courage to listen to that inner voice. As we continue to explore this concept throughout this book, we'll delve deeper into strategies and exercises that can help us connect more closely with our inner wisdom, leading to a more authentic and fulfilling life.

Acknowledging the Existence of Inner Wisdom

Have you ever had that gentle nudge in your gut, that "sixth sense" prompting you to make a certain choice or go a specific route? That, my friend, is inner wisdom - a quiet guide inside us all, waiting patiently to be acknowledged.

Subtle Signs of Inner Wisdom

Inner wisdom often communicates through feelings or instincts. It's that inexplicable sense of "knowing" that something feels right, or conversely, feels wrong. It could be the gut feeling urging you to take a chance on a risky project, or the soft voice whispering caution when you're about to make a hasty decision.

The beauty of inner wisdom is that it's inherently personal and unique to each of us. It may come to you as a sudden insight while in the shower, or perhaps as an intuition about someone you just met.

Practical Tip: Tuning Into Your Inner Wisdom

To better acknowledge your inner wisdom, you need to create the right environment for it to flourish. Find quiet time for reflection and solitude. Meditation, nature walks, or simply sitting quietly can provide the necessary space. When you quiet the noise of the outer world, the voice of your inner world becomes clearer.

Reflections and Acknowledgments

Let's make this concept tangible. Reflect on a decision you made recently where you felt a strong pull towards or against something. What did that feel like? Did you listen? How did the situation unfold as a result? Identifying these instances helps in recognizing the existence of inner wisdom.

Inner wisdom is your personal North Star, a compass guiding you through life's journey. As you learn to acknowledge and trust it, you'll find that you are not wandering aimlessly, but navigating with purpose and clarity. Embrace the inner wisdom within you – it's one of the most empowering things you can do.

Connecting with Your Inner Wisdom through Yoga and Meditation

Allow me to take you on a journey through an ancient practice that opens up a gateway to our inner wisdom: Yoga and meditation. Akin to building a bridge, these practices can provide a direct path to your deepest insights, making the intangible tangible.

The Intersection of Yoga, Meditation, and Inner Wisdom

Imagine your inner wisdom as a quiet river flowing beneath the hustle and bustle of your daily life. Yoga and meditation are like building a well to tap into this river. These practices quiet the noise of the outer world, allowing you to listen to your inner voice.

Yoga promotes mindfulness and self-awareness. Each pose encourages a journey inwards, prompting a silent dialogue between mind and body. Meditation, on the other hand, trains your mind to concentrate and detangle from the web of thoughts, making way for inner wisdom to rise to the surface.

Practical Tip: Postures and Practices for Inner Connection

Begin with yoga asanas (poses) that promote introspection, such as Child's Pose (Balasana), Seated Forward Bend (Paschimottanasana), and Lotus Pose (Padmasana). These poses stimulate the parasympathetic nervous system, fostering a state of relaxation and openness.

In meditation, you can start with a simple mindfulness practice. Sit comfortably, focus on your breath, and let your thoughts flow without engaging with them. Over time, you'll notice the emergence of a clearer, calmer inner voice.

A Guided Meditation to Connect with Inner Wisdom

Now, let's try a guided meditation.

1. Find a peaceful spot and sit comfortably, either on a chair or cross-legged on the floor.
2. Close your eyes and take deep, calming breaths. Feel the sensation of breath entering and leaving your body.
3. Visualize a soft, glowing light at your core. This represents your inner wisdom.
4. Allow this light to expand with each breath, illuminating your whole being.
5. Ask yourself a question you've been pondering. Allow the question to float in your mind.
6. Listen. Your inner wisdom may respond immediately, or it may take some time. Be patient.
7. Once you've spent some time in silence, gently bring your awareness back to your physical surroundings.

Remember, accessing your inner wisdom is not a one-time event but a process. Yoga and meditation are tools that, when used consistently, can help you tune in to your inner voice more effectively. They are bridges to your inner wisdom, waiting to be crossed.

Recognizing the Signs of Inner Wisdom and Cultivating a Sense of Inner Peace to Access Your Inner Wisdom

Picture this: a still lake, untroubled by the wind, reflecting the tranquillity of a serene sky. This is the state of inner peace, the fertile ground where the seeds of inner wisdom can sprout and flourish.

I remember my first experience with this feeling of inner peace. It was during a silent retreat in the tranquil hills of Colorado. As I sat on the edge of a still lake, I experienced a sense of peace I had never felt before. It was a clear, calm state of mind, just like the still lake in front of me. It was then that I realized this calmness is the environment in which our inner wisdom can truly come alive.

Recognizing the Echo of Inner Wisdom

The voice of inner wisdom often comes softly, a whisper amidst the clamor of our everyday thoughts. It can manifest as a gut feeling, an intuition, or a sudden flash of insight. Inner wisdom is patient, non-judgmental, and always in harmony with your true self. However, its gentle voice can be drowned out by the cacophony of our fears, doubts, and worries.

Identifying your inner wisdom involves differentiating it from these distracting voices. This discernment is a skill that needs cultivation, and its mastery can dramatically transform your life. The more you learn to recognize these signs of inner wisdom, the more confidently you can navigate your life, secure in the knowledge that you're aligned with your deepest truths. Let's discuss how this can be applied on a practical level.

Practical Tip: Cultivating Inner Peace and Recognizing Inner Wisdom

Nurturing inner peace is like tending to that still lake. To achieve this, we can practice mindfulness, gratitude, yoga, and meditation. These techniques not only lower stress, but they also create a setting where your inner wisdom can flourish.

Begin by setting aside quiet time each day for self-reflection. You might spend this time in meditation, immersing yourself in nature, or journaling. Pay attention to recurring themes, feelings, or thoughts that come up during these times.

Additionally, consciously limit your exposure to negative influences that can disrupt your inner peace. This may include news media, negative people, or stressful situations.

In my own journey, I found that limiting my exposure to negative news and distancing myself from individuals who drained my energy made a significant difference. It helped to maintain my inner peace, allowing my inner wisdom to shine through more readily.

After mastering recognizing your inner wisdom through journaling, the next step is nurturing it, allowing it to guide you further.

Journaling to Recognize Inner Wisdom

You've become quite proficient with your journal, I see. Let's continue using it to facilitate recognizing your inner wisdom. Here are some prompts for your exploration:

1. Reflect on a time when you experienced a "gut feeling" or intuition that guided you in a certain direction. What was the situation? How did this feeling manifest?
2. Do you recall a situation where you ignored your inner wisdom? What were the consequences? In hindsight, can you identify the voice of your inner wisdom?
3. Describe the voice or feeling of your inner wisdom. How does it differ from other thoughts or feelings?
4. Write about a decision you need to make. After quieting your mind, ask your inner wisdom for guidance. What does it tell you?

Remember, cultivating inner peace and recognizing your inner wisdom is an ongoing journey, not a destination. It's about becoming a gardener of the soul, patiently tending to the stillness within, creating the perfect environment for your inner wisdom to grow and flourish. And as you continue on this path, you'll find the voice of your inner wisdom becomes louder and clearer, guiding you towards a life that is truly in alignment with your deepest self.

Having understood how journaling aids in recognizing our inner wisdom, let's now delve deeper into how this practice nurtures our inner wisdom.

Nurturing Your Inner Wisdom and Using Journaling to Tap into Your Inner Wisdom

Just as we nurture a garden, ensuring it gets the right amount of sun, water, and nutrients, we can also cultivate our inner wisdom. We feed it with awareness, stillness, and reflection, allowing it to grow and flourish. Journaling is an exceptional tool that can help in this cultivation process, creating a fertile ground where inner wisdom can take root.

Tending the Garden of Inner Wisdom

Your inner wisdom is a seed waiting to be nurtured. It requires specific conditions to thrive: an open heart, a calm mind, and a willingness to listen deeply. But how can we create these conditions and foster our inner wisdom?

First, develop a practice of silence and solitude. This can be as simple as spending a few quiet moments each day in meditation or reflection. It's during these moments of silence that we can hear the whisper of our inner wisdom.

Second, cultivate self-awareness. Pay attention to your feelings, thoughts, and experiences. Recognize patterns, acknowledge your feelings without judgment, and understand how they guide your reactions and decisions. Being aware of yourself is like the sunlight that nourishes your inner wisdom.

Lastly, be patient. Just like a gardener doesn't expect a seed to sprout overnight, inner wisdom unfolds in its own time. With patience and perseverance, the subtle voice within you will grow louder and clearer.

Having established the steps to nurture your inner wisdom, let's explore how journaling can become a practical tool in this endeavor.

Practical Tip: Journaling Your Way to Inner Wisdom

You have already built a solid foundation with journaling in the previous chapters. Let's delve deeper into how this practice can help you tap into your inner wisdom.

Start by creating a sacred space for your journaling. Find a quiet spot where you won't be disturbed. This will be your sanctuary for self-reflection and discovery.

Write consistently. Aim to write a few lines every day. It's not about quantity but about establishing a routine that allows you to connect with your inner self.

Use your journal to document your thoughts, feelings, dreams, and fears, but also the intuitive nudges and 'aha' moments. These are the signals of your inner wisdom. Over time, you'll begin to see patterns and discover your unique inner wisdom language.

Don't censor or judge your thoughts. Let your writing flow naturally. This raw, uncensored dialogue with your inner self helps uncover your deepest insights.

Now that we have understood the way to journal for inner wisdom, let's delve into some specific prompts that can guide you in your journaling journey.

Journaling Prompts for Nurturing Inner Wisdom

Let's continue with your journaling practice. Here are some prompts to inspire your exploration:

1. What is one intuitive nudge you've felt recently? How did it manifest? How did you respond?
2. Reflect on a decision you made solely based on your intuition. What was the outcome?
3. Write a conversation between your inner critic and your inner wisdom. What do they say?

I recall one particular entry in my journal where my inner critic was loud and harsh, criticizing a decision I'd made. But then, my inner wisdom gently intervened, reminding me of my strengths and the lessons I'd learned. It was a revealing conversation and a powerful testament to the balance between self-criticism and self-acceptance.

4. How has listening to your inner wisdom changed your life? If you're just beginning, how do you envision your life changing as you cultivate your inner wisdom?

Like a mirror reflecting our deepest selves, journaling can illuminate our path to inner wisdom. It offers a tangible way to access, understand, and nurture the subtle voice within. As you continue on this journey of self-discovery and inner wisdom cultivation, remember the words of wisdom from Lao Tzu: Deep inside, you have the answers; you know your true self and what you desire.

As you explore these journaling prompts, you will deepen your understanding of your inner wisdom. But remember, a crucial aspect of nurturing your inner wisdom involves being open to new perspectives and insights.

While journaling can assist us in recognizing and nurturing our inner wisdom, it is equally essential to remain open to the new insights that this wisdom may present.

Being Open to New Perspectives and Insights from Your Inner Wisdom

The journey to inner wisdom is filled with unexpected turns, revelations, and novel insights. It's crucial to remain open and flexible, embracing new perspectives that challenge our assumptions and help us grow. This section will explore the importance of openness in harnessing inner wisdom and provide techniques for cultivating an open mindset.

I remember an instance when I encountered a perspective that completely contradicted my existing beliefs. At first, I was resistant, but with time and openness, I realized it offered me a broader understanding of the world and myself.

Embracing the Unknown

As we tap into our inner wisdom, we may encounter ideas that seem unfamiliar or even uncomfortable. It's natural to feel resistant, but remaining open to these fresh perspectives allows us to evolve, heal, and gain a deeper understanding of ourselves.

Being open to new insights is an invitation to growth, leading us to question our long-held beliefs, values, and attitudes. As we embrace these new perspectives, we create a richer, more complex inner landscape that expands our understanding of ourselves and the world.

While embracing the unknown might feel daunting, it is an integral part of cultivating an open mindset.

Practical Tip: Cultivating Openness

Cultivating an open mindset requires practice and intention. Here are some techniques to help you foster this mindset:

1. Suspend judgment: Approach your inner wisdom with curiosity and a non-judgmental attitude. Give yourself permission to explore new ideas, even if they challenge your existing beliefs.
2. Embrace uncertainty: Life is full of uncertainties, and that's where growth happens. Allow yourself to be comfortable with not having all the answers and trust that your inner wisdom will guide you through the unknown.
3. Practice mindfulness: Mindfulness involves being fully present in the moment and accepting whatever arises without judgment. This helps create space for new insights and perspectives to emerge.
4. Seek diverse experiences: Expose yourself to different ideas, cultures, and experiences. This not only makes your life richer but also broadens your worldview and makes you more receptive to fresh insights.

Once you've started cultivating an open mindset, it's important to take a step back and explore how open you actually are to new perspectives.

Exploring Openness to New Perspectives

As you continue to cultivate an open mindset, it's essential to reflect on how receptive you are to new perspectives. Here's a self-reflection exercise to help you explore your openness:

1. Consider a recent situation where you encountered a new idea or perspective that challenged your existing beliefs. Write about the emotions you felt and your initial reaction. Did you resist or embrace the new perspective?
2. What did you learn from this experience? How did this new perspective influence your thinking or actions?
3. Reflect on how open you are to receiving insights from your inner wisdom. On a scale of 1-10 (with 10 being the most open), how open are you to allowing your inner wisdom to guide you in unfamiliar or uncomfortable situations?
4. Identify one area of your life where you feel resistant to new perspectives or change. Write about why you feel this resistance and what steps you can take to cultivate greater openness in this area.

As you continue on your journey to access and nurture your inner wisdom, embrace the opportunity to grow through new perspectives and insights. Remember, the treasure trove of inner wisdom within you is vast and ever-evolving, waiting for you to explore its depths. By cultivating openness, you unlock the door to a world of endless possibilities and personal transformation.

While exploring openness and inner wisdom, it's also crucial to honor our physical boundaries, and for that, yoga offers an excellent path.

While mental and emotional openness is crucial in exploring our inner wisdom, we should not forget the physical aspect of our existence. Yoga provides an excellent path for this.

Yoga Poses for Honoring Your Limits and Listening to Your Body

Yoga is a powerful practice that not only strengthens the body but also deepens our connection with it. A key aspect of yoga is honoring our limits, respecting our boundaries, and learning to listen when our body speaks. Here, we will discuss specific yoga poses that facilitate this deeper connection, enhance body awareness, and encourage us to honor our personal boundaries.

Understanding Your Body Through Yoga

Each of our bodies is unique, with its own strengths, limitations, and ways of expressing itself. Yoga encourages us to tap into this innate body wisdom, helping us understand and respect our individual boundaries.

In my own yoga practice, I've discovered the importance of listening to my body. One day, while pushing into a difficult pose, I felt a strain. Instead of forcing it, I honored my body's signal to pull back. It was a lesson in respecting my body's limits and acknowledging its wisdom.

By consciously tuning into our body's signals during yoga, we learn to decipher its language, identifying our comfort zones, points of resistance, and areas where we can safely push a little further.

Practical Tip: Balasana (Child's Pose)

Child's pose, or Balasana, is a resting pose often used to reconnect with the breath, ground ourselves, and honor our body's need for rest. Here's how to do it:

- Kneel on your mat with your big toes touching and sit on your heels.
- Separate your knees about hip-width apart.
- Exhale and lay your torso down between your thighs, extending your arms along the mat, palms facing down.
- Rest your forehead on the mat and breathe deeply.

Allow this pose to be your safe space, returning to it anytime you need to listen to your body's signals and honor its need for rest.

Salamba Sirsasana (Supported Headstand)

- While a more advanced pose, the Supported Headstand, or Salamba Sirsasana, provides a unique opportunity to honor your limits and listen to your body. This pose requires strength, balance, and a careful attention to your body's signals. It's important not to rush into this pose if you're not ready - this is where honoring your limits comes in. If you do feel ready, here's a simple guide:
- Start on all fours, then interlace your fingers and place your forearms on the mat.
- Rest your head between your hands.
- Walk your feet towards your elbows, lifting your hips.
- When ready, gently lift your feet off the mat.
- Engage your core, keeping your legs straight and aligned with your body.

Remember, practicing yoga is not about perfecting poses but about the journey of self-exploration. Listen to your body, respect its messages, and don't push yourself into a pose if it doesn't feel right. Always practice with mindfulness, patience, and self-compassion.

Practical Tip: Marjaryasana-Bitilasana (Cat-Cow Pose)

The Cat-Cow pose is a simple yet effective yoga pose that enhances body awareness and helps us tune into our physical limits. Here's how to do it:

- Start on all fours with your wrists directly under your shoulders and your knees under your hips.
- As you inhale, drop your belly towards the mat, lift your chin and chest, and gaze up towards the ceiling (Cow pose).
- As you exhale, draw your belly to your spine and round your back towards the ceiling (Cat pose).
- Repeat this movement with your breath.

This pose invites us to move with our breath and listen to our body's rhythm, enhancing our connection with our inner self.

Tadasana (Mountain Pose)

Tadasana, or Mountain pose, may seem simple, but it's a powerful pose for grounding and tuning into your body. Here's how to perform this pose:

- Stand tall on your yoga mat, with your feet hip-width apart and your weight evenly distributed between them.
- Relax your shoulders, lengthen your spine, and reach the crown of your head toward the sky, grounding your feet into the earth.
- Place your hands down by your sides, palms facing forward to open your chest.
- Close your eyes and take deep, steady breaths, focusing on the sensation of your feet connecting with the ground and the movement of breath in your body.

This pose invites us to feel grounded and stable, reminding us to remain present and connected with our body's innate wisdom. The simplicity of the Mountain Pose allows for inner reflection and openness to our body's subtle signals.

Practical Tip: Savasana (Corpse Pose)

Savasana, or Corpse Pose, may be the most crucial part of any yoga practice. It's a restorative pose that allows your body and mind to process and integrate the benefits of your practice. Here's how to do it:

- Lie flat on your back, arms at your sides, palms up.

- Allow your legs to fall naturally apart.
- Close your eyes and take slow, deep breaths.
- Relax your body into the mat, releasing tension from each part of your body, starting from your toes and moving up to the crown of your head.

Remain in this pose for at least five minutes, letting go of all effort in your breath and body. Savasana is the perfect pose to honor your limits, acknowledging the work you've done and allowing your body to rest and rejuvenate.

Remember, each yoga pose presents an opportunity to honor your body's limits and listen to its wisdom. Pay attention to the messages your body sends you during your practice, adjusting your movements to accommodate your comfort and safety. It's not about how the pose looks, but how it feels. Embrace your journey, respect your pace, and remember - yoga is a practice of self-love and acceptance, not competition or comparison.

Guided Meditation: Connecting with Your Inner Wisdom

Learning to listen to your inner wisdom is akin to learning a new language, the language of the soul. Meditation serves as a translator, allowing your conscious mind to understand the subtle whispers of your deep intuitive self. Here, I'll guide you through a simple meditation practice to aid in this spiritual translation.

Preparation: Creating a Conducive Environment

Practical Tip: You may find your meditation practice more enjoyable and effective in a quiet, peaceful setting. Create a space in your home specifically for meditation, free from distractions and noise. You might consider adding elements that engage your senses and promote relaxation, such as a comfortable cushion, calming music, or a diffuser with soothing essential oils.

Settle into your meditation spot at a time when you won't be interrupted. Before starting, ensure that you're in comfortable clothing and consider turning off your phone or any other potential distractions.

Step-by-Step Guided Meditation

1. **Finding your Seat:** Sit comfortably on your cushion or chair, ensuring your spine is straight but not tense. Rest your hands gently on your lap. If you prefer, this meditation can also be done lying down.

2. **Focus on your Breath:** Close your eyes and begin to tune into your breath. Notice the rise and fall of your chest and abdomen as you breathe in and out. Don't try to change your breathing; simply observe it.
3. **Body Scan:** Starting from the crown of your head and moving down to your toes, mentally scan your body. As you do this, notice any areas of tension or discomfort, then use your breath to release this tension on every exhale.
4. **Inviting your Inner Wisdom:** Visualize a soft, glowing light in the center of your chest. This light represents your inner wisdom. See it grow brighter with each breath. As it illuminates, it brings clarity, guidance, and peace.
5. **Ask and Listen:** Silently ask a question that you'd like guidance on. It can be a simple or complex question, about a current situation or a broader aspect of your life. After asking, return to the silence, the space that lies between your thoughts, and listen.
6. **Trust the Process:** Remember, your inner wisdom might not always speak in clear, distinct words. Its guidance can also come in the form of feelings, images, or subtle gut instincts. Trust the process and know that your intuition is sending you the right messages, even if you don't fully understand them at the moment.
7. **Closing the Practice:** When you feel ready, bring your awareness back to your physical surroundings. Wiggle your fingers and toes, and when you're ready, slowly open your eyes. Sit quietly for a few moments to assimilate the experience before getting up .

In this meditative state, your mind is calm and clear, providing fertile ground for the seeds of intuition to take root and flourish. Use this guided meditation as a tool to nurture your relationship with your inner wisdom, cultivating a deeper understanding of yourself and your path. Regular practice will foster an ongoing dialogue with your intuitive self, illuminating the wise inner guidance that is always available to you

Inner Wisdom Vision Board

Let's explore an exciting, tactile tool for manifesting your inner wisdom: the Vision Board. Traditionally used as a visualization tool for goals and dreams, we can adapt it to our purpose of harnessing inner wisdom.

Understanding the Vision Board

A Vision Board is a visual representation of your aspirations. In our context, it's an external, tangible canvas reflecting your inner wisdom. It helps give form to and anchor the intuitive insights and nudges you experience, making them more tangible and easier to understand.

Just as a map aids a traveler in their journey, your Vision Board can guide you in your personal growth, shedding light on your path and providing clarity and motivation.

Practical Tip: Crafting Your Inner Wisdom Vision Board

Creating an Inner Wisdom Vision Board is a delightful, creative process. Here's a step-by-step guide:

Step 1: Gather Your Materials - You'll need a board (like cork or poster board), glue, scissors, and an assortment of magazines, printed images, or words.

Step 2: Set the Mood - Find a peaceful space and time where you can dive into this process without interruption. You may wish to light a candle, play soothing music, or create an atmosphere that feels comforting.

Step 3: Reflection - Spend a few moments in quiet contemplation. Connect with your inner wisdom, recalling the insights you've gained through meditation, journaling, or simple introspection.

Step 4: Visual Representation - Begin to seek images, words, or symbols that represent these insights and guidance from your inner wisdom. Be intuitive and spontaneous in your selection. Cut these out.

Step 5: Assemble Your Vision Board - Start arranging your chosen elements on your board. There's no right or wrong here. Trust your instinct, allowing your board to unfold organically. Once you're satisfied with your layout, glue the elements down.

Step 6: Position for Reflection - Place your Vision Board somewhere you'll see it regularly. It will serve as a visual reminder of the profound wisdom within you, keeping it at the forefront of your consciousness.

Consider your Inner Wisdom Vision Board as a dynamic reflection of your evolving journey. As you grow and uncover more layers of your inner wisdom, feel free to modify the board accordingly. Embrace this process as a joyous exercise of creativity and introspection.

The Power of Honoring Your Inner Wisdom

In this chapter, we've embarked on a transformative journey, exploring the vast, radiant world within us, nurturing our inner wisdom, and employing powerful tools such as journaling, yoga, and meditation.

Reflecting on my own journey, I recall a time in my life when I faced a challenging situation, torn between the expected and the uncertain. It was my inner wisdom that guided me to trust my intuition and choose the path less traveled. The journey wasn't easy, but it led me to a realization of my true potential and the beauty of authenticity. This personal experience reinforced the value of honoring and trusting my inner wisdom.

As you incorporate these practices into your life, remember that patience and consistency are key. It's not merely about reaching an endpoint but rather appreciating the journey itself. Continue to cultivate a nurturing environment for your inner wisdom to flourish, and don't shy away from revisiting or refining these practices as you grow and change.

Reflective Questions:

1. What insights have emerged from your journaling practice so far?
2. How does incorporating yoga into your daily routine make you feel?

3. What messages have you received from your inner wisdom during your meditation practice?

4. How has creating an Inner Wisdom Vision Board helped make your intuitions more tangible?

5. In what ways has honoring your inner wisdom influenced your daily life?

As we look forward to the next chapter, 'Owning Your Power,' we will delve into the strength that lies within you and learn how to harness it effectively. We will explore how yoga and personal growth can amplify your personal power, and understand the role of self-care and boundary-setting in owning your power. There will be tips, exercises, and interactive elements to guide you along the way.

Before we leap into the next chapter, I invite you to spend some time reflecting on the insights you've gained so far. Practice a yoga pose, or begin gathering materials for your Inner Wisdom Vision Board.

This journey towards self-discovery isn't a sprint; it's a marathon, where each step represents a personal victory, no matter how small it may seem. It's about savoring the process, the lessons, and the insights you collect along the way.

Remember that growth often comes from the most uncomfortable places. Don't shy away from discomfort; embrace it. Understand that it's okay to feel confused or lost sometimes, as these feelings are just signposts indicating that there's room for growth and learning. It's these experiences that contribute to your resilience, strength, and ultimately, your wisdom.

Self-discovery and personal growth are continuous processes. They require consistent efforts and time to cultivate. While it may feel overwhelming at times, remember that every single step you take is leading you closer to understanding and aligning with your authentic self. Keep faith in your journey and trust your inner wisdom; it's your most reliable guide.

Thank you for joining me in this chapter. I hope you found it enlightening and empowering. I'm excited for what the next chapter holds for you as we explore owning your power, asserting your boundaries, and embracing the strength within you.

May you continue to shine your light brightly, trusting your inner wisdom and harnessing it to lead you towards a more fulfilling and authentic life.

11

Owning Your Power

Welcome, dear reader, to the next exciting juncture of our journey together. We're poised to embark on a profound exploration of your personal power, an aspect of self-discovery and growth that's as vital as it is often overlooked.

Personal Power: A Beacon of Authenticity

In the context of yoga and personal growth, personal power, or 'Manipura', represents your core self, your inner drive, and your ability to assert your space in this world. Your personal power is like your inner compass, guiding you towards your true north amidst the tempests of life. It's your source of courage, resilience, and determination. Owning your power doesn't imply overpowering others; rather, it means standing your ground, living authentically, and making decisions that align with your core beliefs and values.

Your Power, Your Yoga

In yoga, the asanas, or postures, aren't merely physical exercises—they're opportunities to assert your personal power, to be wholly present in your body, and to honor your limits while challenging yourself to grow. As we delve deeper into this chapter, we'll examine how different yoga poses can help you cultivate and harness your personal power.

Power Perception Quiz

Before we go further, it's essential to understand where you currently stand in your perception of personal power. So, I invite you to participate in a brief self-assessment quiz. This activity aims to offer a snapshot of your current relationship with your personal power and serve as a baseline as we move forward. Please take this as a reflective exercise, rather than a test. There are no right or wrong answers here—only insights about your journey.

1. How would you describe your level of confidence in your abilities?

    A. Very high - I believe in my skills and capabilities

    B. Somewhat high - I generally believe in myself, but sometimes I doubt

    C. Average - I have faith in some areas, but not in others

    D. Low - I frequently doubt my abilities

2. When faced with a difficult situation, do you believe you have the power to influence the outcome?

    A. Always - I believe I can affect change in any circumstance

    B. Most of the time - I feel that I can often make a difference

    C. Sometimes - I feel I can influence some situations but not others

    D. Rarely - I usually feel like things are out of my control

3. How often do you assert yourself in personal and professional settings?

    A. Always - I am confident and make my voice heard

    B. Often - I assert myself when I feel it's important

    C. Sometimes - I find it difficult to assert myself in certain situations

    D. Rarely - I struggle to assert myself and express my thoughts

4. Do you feel comfortable taking risks and trying new things?

    A. Yes, always - I embrace new challenges and experiences

    B. Most of the time - I like trying new things, but sometimes I hesitate

    C. Sometimes - I can be hesitant and require some encouragement

D. Rarely - I tend to avoid risks and prefer sticking to what I know

5. How do you react when you make a mistake or fail at something?

A. I view it as a learning opportunity and grow from the experience

B. I get upset initially, but then try to learn from it

C. I tend to dwell on it and struggle to move past it

D. I often feel defeated and question my abilities

Depending on the responses:

Mostly As: You have a strong sense of personal power. You are confident in your abilities and generally feel that you have the power to influence your life's direction.

Mostly Bs: You have a good sense of personal power, but there may be areas where you lack confidence. You sometimes question your ability to effect change but generally believe in yourself.

Mostly Cs: You may have a moderate sense of personal power, but there might be situations where you feel less confident or in control. It may be beneficial to focus on building your confidence and belief in your abilities.

Mostly Ds: You may struggle with feeling powerful and confident in yourself. This is okay, and it's a starting point. It shows that there is room for growth and self-improvement.

Remember, personal power is a journey, not a destination. As you continue to learn and grow, your sense of personal power can evolve and expand.

The upcoming lessons in this chapter are geared towards embracing your personal power, nurturing your self-esteem, and helping you navigate through life with confidence and assertion. Let's courageously delve into the realm of personal power, embarking on a new chapter of growth and self-discovery.

Remember, as we traverse this new terrain, keep your inner wisdom close. Trust it. It has guided you this far and it will continue to light your way as you dive deeper into the exploration of your personal power. Here's to asserting your boundaries, owning your power, and embracing the strength within you.

This journey is yours, and every step forward is a testament to your resilience. Keep shining your light brightly. Your adventure towards a more fulfilling and authentic life continues.

Understanding Personal Power

The essence of personal power is often misunderstood and misconstrued. It's not about imposing your will on others or being 'in control'. Personal power is about inner strength, resilience, and autonomy. It's about owning your space, taking responsibility for your actions, and making conscious decisions that align with your values and goals.

Different Aspects of Personal Power

Personal power takes shape through various aspects of our lives. Firstly, it manifests as self-confidence, a belief in one's abilities and worth. Secondly, it's seen in assertiveness, the capacity to express your needs and stand up for your rights respectfully. Thirdly, personal power is about resilience, the strength to weather adversity and bounce back. Lastly, it's about autonomy, the ability to act independently and make decisions based on personal judgment.

Personal Power in Daily Life

To illustrate, let me share a personal story. Once, during a particularly challenging yoga class, I found myself struggling with a complex pose. My body was trembling, sweat was trickling down my face, and a part of me wanted to give up. But then, I heard a voice in my head, saying, "You've got this." I took a deep breath, focused on my core, and managed to hold the pose, albeit imperfectly. I realized then that my personal power didn't lie in executing the pose flawlessly, but in the courage to persist, the resilience to endure, and the autonomy to choose to continue despite the discomfort.

This moment was a microcosm of how personal power can manifest in our lives. Whether it's holding a challenging yoga pose, navigating a tricky situation at work, or overcoming personal hardship, our personal power serves as our guiding light.

Reflecting on Personal Power

Now, I invite you to reflect on your own experiences.

1. When have you experienced a boost in your self-confidence?
2. Can you recall a moment where you asserted yourself respectfully?
3. How have you demonstrated resilience in the face of adversity?
4. When have you felt autonomous, making a decision solely based on your judgment?

These questions aren't about judging or grading your personal power but about recognising its presence in your life. Reflection is a powerful tool to uncover insights that might otherwise remain hidden.

As we continue our journey, remember that understanding and owning your personal power is an evolving process. Your personal power is not static; it grows and matures with you. Cultivating it is like tending a garden: you plant the seeds, nourish them, provide the right conditions for growth, and with patience, you'll see them bloom.

In the next sections, we'll delve deeper into harnessing and strengthening your personal power. As always, trust your journey and believe in the wisdom within you. Your path towards a more fulfilling and authentic life is yours to forge.

The Yoga Practice for Empowerment

Yoga, as we've explored throughout this journey, is far more than just a physical practice. It's an intricate dance of body, mind, and spirit—a tool for empowerment that can help us realize our personal power and draw it forth with grace and purpose.

Yoga as a Pathway to Empowerment

Physically, yoga invites us to challenge our bodies, fostering strength, resilience, and a deep sense of embodiment. But it's the mental and emotional aspects of yoga that are truly transformative. Through mindful movement, focused breathing, and deep meditation, yoga becomes a mirror reflecting our inner selves. It teaches us about our limits and potential, about the courage to try, the resilience to endure, and the wisdom to rest.

Practical Tip: Setting Up an Empowering Yoga Practice

As you step onto your mat, remember that an empowering yoga practice begins with intention. Before you start, take a moment to set an intention that resonates with your need for personal power. It could be as simple as "I am strong," or as specific as "I trust my ability to navigate this challenge."

Choose poses that encourage a sense of empowerment, like the Warrior sequence, which embodies strength and determination, or the Mountain pose, representing steadiness and grounding. In each pose, visualize your personal power as a golden light within you, expanding with each inhale, grounding you with each exhale.

A Guided Visualization Exercise

Now, let's further enhance your yoga practice with a guided visualization exercise. Close your eyes and take a few deep breaths. Visualize yourself standing at the edge of a beautiful, tranquil lake. The water is perfectly still, reflecting the calm, peaceful sky above.

As you step onto your yoga mat in this tranquil setting, you see a golden orb of light at your core. This light represents your personal power. With each breath, each pose, the light grows brighter, stronger, illuminating the path you're about to take on your mat. As you navigate through your practice, the light continues to glow, a beacon of strength, resilience, and autonomy.

After your practice, carry this visualization with you, off the mat and into your daily life. Let this radiant light of personal power guide you, reminding you of your inner strength and resilience.

Through the practice of yoga and visualization, we can nurture and empower our personal power, turning it into a driving force for growth and transformation. As you continue to evolve on your journey towards self-discovery, remember to keep your light shining brightly, illuminating your path towards a more fulfilling, authentic life.

Building Physical Strength through Yoga

Physical strength is an intrinsic part of personal power. The belief in our physical capabilities empowers us, giving us the confidence to face life's challenges head-on. Yoga, with its blend of flexibility, balance, and strength training, can be an invaluable tool in this journey towards physical empowerment.

To illustrate this concept, I would like to share my personal journey with yoga. I've found yoga to be a transformative practice, significantly enhancing my physical strength and overall confidence. Starting as a beginner, struggling to maintain even the most basic poses, I've witnessed a profound change in my physical abilities over time. This experience, filled with small victories and constant learning, has given me the courage to face life's challenges with a renewed sense of power and belief in myself.

The Power of Yoga: Physical Strength and Beyond

Yoga poses, or 'asanas', require us to engage multiple muscle groups simultaneously, fostering holistic strength. It isn't about isolating and building one muscle group; it's about creating an interconnected web of strength throughout your body. This physical strength not only benefits us in our daily tasks but also enhances our sense of personal power, giving us the confidence to assert ourselves and the resilience to overcome physical and emotional challenges.

But the benefits of yoga don't stop at physical strength. The mindfulness in movement required in yoga helps us tune into our bodies, increasing our body awareness.

This heightened awareness can lead to improved posture, better movement patterns, and a greater appreciation for our physical capabilities, further boosting our personal power. According to a study published in the Journal of Physical Activity and Health, regular yoga practice can improve balance and mobility, as well as increase body awareness (Smith et al., 2013).

Now that we've discussed the theoretical benefits of yoga, let's delve into some practical applications.

Practical Tip: Strength-Building Yoga Poses and Sequences

My Personal Journey with the Warrior Sequence

Let me share a personal experience that really illustrates the transformative power of yoga. When I first embarked on my yoga journey, the Warrior Sequence seemed like an insurmountable challenge. In particular, the Warrior III pose tested my limits. I remember the frustration of wobbling, the embarrassment of losing my balance, and the feeling of defeat as I struggled to lift my back leg. But I stuck with it. Each day was an emotional rollercoaster, filled with small victories and setbacks. With every wobble, I found new reserves of determination. With each held pose, a wave of triumph washed over me. Little by little, I could feel myself getting stronger, more stable. It was a slow process, but over time, not only did I master the pose, but I also felt more powerful and capable in other aspects of my life. It's this holistic transformation, the strengthening of both body and mind, that makes yoga such an empowering practice.

Now let's delve into some specific yoga poses and sequences that can help you build physical strength.

> **Warrior Sequence:** This series, including Warrior I, II, and III, is fantastic for building strength in your legs, core, and shoulders. It also fosters mental resilience and focus.

The Warrior Sequence, steeped in ancient lore, is said to represent the spiritual warrior battling the universal enemy, self-ignorance, the ultimate source of all our suffering. Each pose embodies a different aspect of this spiritual struggle, embodying the strength, focus, and determination it requires

Imagine standing firm on the ground, with one foot facing forward and the other at a 90-degree angle. Your body is stretched tall, and your arms are reaching out in a straight line, with your gaze set on your front hand. This is the Warrior II pose, a symbol of strength and concentration.

Just like the Warrior II pose, each asana in yoga has a rich backstory and symbolism. For instance, the Tree Pose, while looking simple, symbolizes stability and grounding, drawing from the unwavering strength and deep roots of trees. Meanwhile, the Plank Pose, a highly physical pose, represents resilience and endurance, mirroring the firmness of a wooden plank. Sharing the stories behind these asanas will allow readers to appreciate their deeper meaning and philosophy, and might inspire them to approach the practice with a more spiritual perspective.

> **Plank Pose:** Holding a plank not only strengthens your arms, shoulders, and core but also improves endurance.

> **Tree Pose:** While this might look simple, balancing on one leg strengthens your ankles and calves and engages your core.

Bridge Pose: This asana works your glutes, back, and inner thighs. It's also a heart-opening pose, promoting emotional strength.

Boat Pose: Perfect for engaging and strengthening your entire core.

Consider incorporating these poses into your regular yoga practice. Remember, it's not about how long you can hold a pose, but the quality of your form and your mindful engagement with the pose.

In yoga, every pose is an opportunity to build strength and personal power. But remember, strength in yoga isn't just about the physical—it's also about mental resilience and emotional balance. As you move through these strength-building poses, hold onto your inner wisdom, use it as a source of guidance and motivation. Remember to listen to your body, to respect its limits and to celebrate its progress.

After understanding the specific poses, it's also beneficial to familiarize yourself with different styles of yoga, as they offer varying experiences and benefits

Different styles of yoga offer different experiences and benefits. Hatha Yoga, for instance, is slower-paced and more focused on holding poses, which can build strength and flexibility. Ashtanga and Power Yoga are faster-paced and more challenging, offering a more intense strength-building workout.

As we've seen throughout this chapter, owning your personal power is an ongoing journey, one that requires consistent effort and nurturing. By harnessing the transformative power of yoga, we can all inch closer to a more empowered, authentic version of ourselves.

Be patient, be persistent, and above all, be kind to yourself as you navigate this path towards personal empowerment.

While physical strength is a crucial aspect, mental resilience forms an equally, if not more, critical facet of personal power. Let's explore this aspect next.

Developing Mental Resilience through Yoga

Mental resilience, cultivated through yoga, can lead to a profound emotional transformation. It equips us with the inner strength to weather life's storms, to rise again after we've been knocked down, and to find optimism in even the darkest situations. It's this emotional resilience that becomes an unshakable foundation of our personal power. One of the many gifts of yoga is its potential to foster this mental resilience, strengthening our inner resolve and equipping us to navigate life's ups and downs more smoothly.

Yoga and Mental Resilience: A Dynamic Duo

Yoga does more than enhance our physical strength and flexibility; it helps us cultivate a mindset of resilience. By staying present through discomfort, maintaining balance amidst instability, and finding stillness within movement, we learn valuable lessons that apply not just on the mat but in life too. In fact, the mat becomes a microcosm for life itself, allowing us to practice and foster resilience in a safe, controlled environment.

In fact, the mat becomes a microcosm for life itself, allowing us to practice and foster resilience in a safe, controlled environment. Research in the Journal of Psychiatric Practice suggests that yoga can significantly reduce symptoms of depression, anxiety, and stress (Uebelacker et al., 2017).

Let's take balancing poses, for example. Falling out of a pose can be frustrating, but it's also an opportunity to build resilience. Each time we fall and get back up, we reinforce our ability to recover from setbacks. We understand that it's not about perfection, but the journey of learning, growing, and trying again.

Practical Tip: Fostering Mental Resilience through Mindfulness and Meditation

As yoga nurtures our physical strength, meditation and mindfulness practices nurture our mental resilience. Mindfulness encourages us to stay present, non-judgmentally observing our thoughts and feelings without getting swept away by them. This observational stance helps us respond rather than react to life's stressors, fostering resilience.

Consider incorporating mindfulness into your yoga practice. Focus on your breath, the sensations in your body, the ebb and flow of your thoughts. This presence can create a sense of calm and clarity, even amidst challenging poses.

In addition to mindfulness, consider a daily meditation practice. Even just a few minutes a day can significantly improve mental resilience. As you sit in silence, simply observe your thoughts as they come and go. Over time, you may notice a shift—a greater sense of peace, a deeper resilience, a more powerful sense of personal power.

Journal Prompts for Reflection on Mental Resilience and Personal Power

As we've seen in previous chapters, journaling can be a potent tool for reflection and growth. Reflecting on our experiences allows us to gain insights into our mental patterns, enhancing our self-understanding and fostering mental resilience.

Here are some journal prompts to facilitate reflection:

1. Recall a challenging yoga pose or sequence. How did you feel during it? How did you handle the discomfort or challenge?
2. Reflect on a challenging situation in your life. How did you respond to it? How did your yoga practice influence your response?
3. What does mental resilience mean to you? How does it contribute to your sense of personal power?
4. Imagine your life with an even stronger sense of mental resilience. What would be different? How would it affect your personal power?

As you explore these prompts, remember that resilience, like personal power, is a journey, not a destination. It's about continually learning, growing, and empowering yourself, both on the mat and off. Yoga offers us a tangible way to foster this resilience, granting us the tools to embrace our personal power fully.

While building mental resilience, it's also essential to consider the practices of self-care and setting boundaries.

Practicing Self-Care and Setting Boundaries

In our pursuit of personal power, it's crucial to remember the importance of self-care and setting boundaries. Often misunderstood or overlooked, these elements are the bedrock of our mental and physical well-being and essential for sustaining our energy and preserving our personal power.

Self-Care: The Fuel for Personal Power

Self-care is a deeply emotional practice. It's about recognizing our own worthiness, addressing our needs with kindness, and taking the time to replenish our energy reserves. It's an act of self-love that deeply nurtures our well-being.

I remember a time when I was so caught up in my daily grind that I completely neglected self-care. My energy levels were low, and I felt disconnected from my own needs. The turning point came when I started incorporating yoga and mindfulness into my daily routine. I began to listen more to my body, understanding its needs and responding with self-care actions like regular sleep, healthy eating, and taking time out to relax. It was a transformative experience that heightened my sense of self-worth and personal power.

It's about ensuring we're not running on empty but rather filled up and ready to face life's challenges and opportunities. When we take care of ourselves, we're not just sustaining our personal power—we're amplifying it.

However, self-care is more than just bubble baths and pampering—it's about tuning into our needs and honoring them. It could be getting enough sleep, nourishing our bodies with healthy foods, maintaining a regular yoga practice, or taking time for hobbies we love.

Practical Tip: Techniques for Practicing Self-Care

As a yoga practitioner, you have a powerful tool for self-care at your disposal. Regular yoga and meditation practice can reduce stress, improve sleep, and contribute to overall well-being.

Beyond that, consider what other practices nourish you. This could be taking a walk in nature, reading a good book, spending time with loved ones, or just enjoying some quiet time alone. Make a list of your self-care activities and ensure to integrate them into your routine.

Just as vital as self-care in this journey is the act of setting boundaries.

Setting Boundaries: The Shield of Personal Power

Setting boundaries is another crucial aspect of maintaining personal power. It involves defining what we're comfortable with and what's unacceptable, and then communicating that to others. By setting boundaries, we honor our needs, protect our energy, and command respect from others.

For years, I struggled with setting boundaries, often over-extending myself to the point of burnout.

A memorable instance was when I agreed to take on a high-intensity project at work while I was already swamped with other tasks. I found it difficult to say 'no', believing that it would reflect poorly on my capabilities. The result was weeks of constant stress, poor sleep, and ultimately, a sense of burnout.

This experience served as a powerful lesson about the importance of respecting my limits and asserting them to others.

The day I decided to prioritize my needs and communicate my boundaries was a game-changer. I realized that saying 'no' was not a sign of weakness, but rather a declaration of self-respect and personal power.

Practical Tip: Techniques for Setting Healthy Boundaries

Start by identifying areas where you feel depleted or stressed—this could signal a boundary has been crossed. Next, define what a healthier boundary might look like. Finally, communicate your boundaries clearly and respectfully, remembering that it's okay to say no and put your needs first.

Remember, it's not about being selfish or rigid—it's about honoring yourself and your personal power.

A Self-Assessment Exercise

To better understand where you might need to set healthier boundaries, consider the following self-assessment exercise:

1. List the relationships or areas of life where you feel drained, stressed, or taken for granted.
2. Reflect on what a healthier boundary might look like in each of these situations.
3. Consider how you might communicate these boundaries in a respectful yet assertive way.
4. Identify potential challenges or resistance you might face, and brainstorm strategies to address them.

As you engage with this exercise, remember: setting boundaries is a practice, not a one-time event. It requires self-awareness, courage, and consistency. But rest assured, each boundary you set is a powerful affirmation of your worth and a testament to your personal power.

By nurturing our self-care and honing our boundary-setting skills, we can better protect our personal power, ensuring we're not just surviving, but truly thriving. In this way, self-care and boundary-setting become more than just strategies—they become acts of self-love and self-respect, essential components of our journey towards personal power.

While yoga can be a powerful tool for strength and resilience, it's important to approach it with care. Always listen to your body, modify poses as needed, and consider working with a certified yoga teacher, especially if you're a beginner or have any health concerns.

Integrating Yoga into Daily Life for Empowerment

When we think of yoga, we often picture ourselves on a mat in a serene studio. While that's an essential part of the practice, yoga's true power lies in its capacity to extend beyond the mat and permeate our daily lives. Let's explore how we can seamlessly integrate yoga into our routines, fostering a heightened sense of empowerment.

Empowerment through Everyday Yoga

The beauty of yoga lies in its universality - it's not just a physical exercise, but a comprehensive life philosophy. By integrating yogic principles and practices into our everyday lives, we can foster a continual sense of harmony, balance, and empowerment.

Practical Tip: Integrating Yoga into Daily Life

To bring yoga off the mat and into your day, consider these practical suggestions:

> **Morning Ritual:** Start your day with a short yoga practice. This could be a few rounds of Sun Salutations or a simple meditation to set your intention for the day.
>
> **Mindful Breaks:** Use breaks during your day for brief yoga stretches or mindful breathing exercises. These can be particularly helpful during stressful moments or long working hours.

Evening Wind-Down: Use restorative yoga poses or a guided yoga Nidra meditation as a part of your bedtime routine to foster a sense of calm and a good night's sleep.

Yogic Eating: Embrace mindful eating, a concept in line with yogic principles. Pay attention to the tastes, textures, and smells of your food, and listen to your body's hunger and fullness cues.

Yoga Philosophy: Apply the teachings of the Yamas and Niyamas, ethical yogic principles, in your interactions and decision-making processes.

Remember, the goal isn't to transform your daily routine into a yoga marathon but to sprinkle yogic elements throughout your day to keep you connected, balanced, and empowered.

Monday: _____

Tuesday: _____

Wednesday: _____

Thursday: _____

Friday: _____

Saturday: _____

Sunday: _____

For each day, fill in the blank with a yoga practice you'd like to integrate, whether it's a morning Sun Salutation, a midday mindful breathing exercise, or an evening yoga Nidra session. Feel free to get creative and consider your daily obligations, energy levels, and personal preferences.

By integrating yoga into your daily life, you're not just stretching your body but expanding your personal power. It's about turning mundane moments into opportunities for mindfulness, balance, and growth. This way, your mat becomes more than just a physical space—it becomes a symbol of empowerment, a testament to your commitment to personal growth and well-being.

Planning Your Yoga Routine

To help integrate yoga into your routine, here's a simple planning tool. Imagine a weekly layout, with spaces to jot down your yoga practices aligned with your regular schedule:

Exercises and Practices for Owning Your Power

The journey to personal empowerment is a unique one, with various practices and exercises facilitating the process. Yoga, in particular, offers a range of poses that can help tap into our intrinsic power. Let's delve into some practices designed to help you cultivate and own your personal power.

Unleashing Power Through Yoga

Yoga has a unique way of unearthing the strength that resides within us. By connecting breath, movement, and intention, we become more attuned to our innate power. The poses we'll explore are accessible and powerful tools to reinforce this connection.

Practical Tip: Power-Owning Yoga Practices

Let's explore some Level 1 poses not covered in the previous chapters:

Warrior II (Virabhadrasana II): A standing pose that cultivates balance, focus, and resilience. It's a symbol of our inner warrior, representing strength, courage, and personal power.

Gate Pose (Parighasana): A side-bending pose that stretches the spine, arms, and hamstrings. This pose encourages openness and expansiveness.

Goddess Pose (Utkata Konasana): A powerful standing pose that ignites the power of the divine feminine within, fostering a sense of strength and resilience.

Remember, consistency is key. Practicing these poses regularly can help you connect with your inner power.

Power-Owning Yoga Sequence

Let's weave these poses into a simple, empowering yoga sequence:

Warm-up with Mountain Pose (Tadasana): Stand tall, breathe deeply, and set an intention of tapping into your personal power.

Transition into Warrior II (Virabhadrasana II): Step your feet wide apart. Turn your right foot out and bend your right knee. Stretch your arms out to the sides, gaze over your right hand, and breathe deeply.

Move into Gate Pose (Parighasana): Kneel on your mat and stretch your right leg out to the right. Reach your right arm down the right leg and extend your left arm overhead. Feel the stretch along your left side.

Step into Goddess Pose (Utkata Konasana): From a wide stance, turn your toes out and bend your knees. Sink your hips down and reach your arms overhead. Feel the strength in your legs and core.

Repeat Warrior II and Gate Pose on the Left Side: Balance your practice by repeating the poses on the other side.

Conclude in Mountain Pose (Tadasana): Finish where you began, standing tall in Mountain pose. Reflect on your strength and resilience.

Use this sequence as a regular practice to help tap into your personal power. Remember to breathe deeply, maintain a mindful presence, and connect with your intention throughout the practice.

Each of these poses offers a unique opportunity to harness your inner strength. They serve as a metaphor for our potential to stand tall amidst challenges, to bend without breaking, and to harness our power, just like the strong warriors, resilient gates, and divine goddesses they represent. Incorporate these practices into your yoga routine and watch your power flourish.

Guided Meditation: Embracing Your Inner Power

Within each of us is a reservoir of power waiting to be tapped into. One effective way to connect with this inner power is through meditation. Let's embark on a guided journey together.

Creating a Sacred Space for Meditation

Before we begin, it's important to create an environment conducive to meditation. Here's a quick practical tip: Choose a quiet space where you won't be disturbed, dim the lights or light a candle to promote a soothing ambiance, and maybe even include some soft background music or nature sounds. Comfort is key, so ensure your seating arrangement allows you to maintain an upright yet relaxed posture.

Step-by-Step Guided Meditation

1. **Setting the Intention:** Close your eyes and take a moment to set an intention. For this meditation, it could be, "I am ready to embrace my inner power."
2. **Body Scan:** Gradually scan your body from your toes to the crown of your head. As you acknowledge each part, release any tension and feel a warm sense of relaxation spreading.
3. **Visualize Your Inner Power:** Imagine a warm, glowing light at the center of your body. This represents your inner power. With each breath, this light expands, filling your entire body.
4. **Embrace Your Power:** As this light expands, feel it imbuing you with strength, resilience, and courage. It's your source of boundless inner power. It's always been there, and you're now tuning into it.
5. **Affirmations:** Silently repeat affirmations that resonate with your intention, such as "I am powerful," or "I embrace my inner strength." Feel the truth of these affirmations permeating every part of your being.
6. **Return to the Present:** When you're ready, gently bring your attention back to your physical surroundings. Slowly open your eyes, taking a moment to feel the effect of the meditation before you stand up.

Remember, your inner power isn't something you need to seek out; it's already within you. This meditation simply serves as a tool to connect with it, to tune into it, and to remind you of your inherent strength. Practice this meditation regularly and watch how it empowers you to embrace the full magnitude of your potential.

Interactive Exercise: Developing a Personal Power Mantra

Mantras can serve as powerful tools in our journey towards self-empowerment. These phrases or sentences, when repeated, can anchor us in our inner power and guide us through life's ups and downs. Let's dive into the process of creating your Personal Power Mantra.

The Power of a Personal Mantra

A personal power mantra is a positive, affirming statement that resonates deeply with your core self. It's something you can turn to when you need a boost of strength, a reminder of your worth, or simply a grounding force in moments of uncertainty.

Crafting Your Personal Power Mantra

A well-crafted personal power mantra will speak to you and your journey. Here's a step-by-step guide to create your mantra:

1. **Reflection:** Spend some time in quiet reflection, considering your values, your strengths, and your aspirations. What are the qualities you most admire in yourself? What attributes would you like to enhance?
2. **Clarity:** Clearly define what you wish to manifest or reinforce through your mantra. It could be a sense of confidence, resilience, compassion, or any attribute that resonates with you.
3. **Creation:** Formulate a sentence that captures your goal. Ensure it's stated in the present tense and uses positive language. For example, instead of saying, "I want to become more confident," you could say, "I am radiating confidence."
4. **Validation:** Say your mantra out loud and pay attention to how it feels. If it resonates, you've found your mantra! If not, modify the words until they feel right.

Interactive Worksheet: Your Personal Power Mantra

Now, it's your turn! Using a worksheet, jot down your reflections from each step. Remember, there's no 'right' or 'wrong' when creating your mantra. It should simply be authentic to you.

> **Reflections:** Write down your key strengths, values, and aspirations.
>
> **Mantra Goal:** What attribute or feeling would you like your mantra to embody?
>
> **Draft Mantras:** Experiment with several phrases, jotting down all possibilities.

Your Personal Power Mantra: Finalize your mantra. Write it down, and place it somewhere visible as a daily reminder of your personal power.

Remember, your Personal Power Mantra is a tool for you to tap into your innate strength. Use it daily, and watch as it infuses your life with a deeper sense of empowerment and confidence.

The Power of Owning Your Personal Power

We've come a long way on this journey of embracing our personal power. From understanding the concept, exploring yoga poses, guided meditation, and crafting your personal power mantra, every step has been towards empowerment and self-love.

The Transformative Potential of Personal Power

Owning your personal power is transformative. It shapes the way you interact with the world, boosts your self-esteem, and guides you to your truth. This transformative journey, as you've discovered in this chapter, is a continuous one, full of self-discovery, growth, and joy.

Inspiration for Continued Empowerment

Take your newly-found strength and let it guide you forward. Continue with the yoga sequences, meditate with your power mantra, and let your inner light shine. Remember, the journey to empowerment doesn't stop here; it evolves, much like you.

Action Plan for Embracing Personal Power

Now, it's time to solidify your learnings into an action plan. How will you continue to nurture your personal power? What yoga practices will you integrate into your daily life? Use the action plan template to outline these steps, creating a roadmap for your continued journey of self-empowerment.

Reflect on this chapter's key points and the benefits of owning your personal power. Consider the transformation you can expect as you continue implementing these practices. How will your life change? How will you change?

Moving Forward

As we conclude this chapter, reflect on how far you've come. Feel proud of the work you've done to embrace your personal power. Remember, every pose, every breath, every mantra is a step towards your true, powerful self.

With your newfound power, I invite you to step into the next chapter, "Beyond the Mat." Here, we'll explore how you can carry these principles of yoga and personal power into your everyday life. From integrating yoga into your daily routines to understanding its role in living a more fulfilling life, we will delve deeper into the transformative journey that is yoga.

So, keep your mat close, your mantra closer, and your mind open to the beautiful transformations that lie ahead. Your journey to self-empowerment continues, and the power within you is ready to shine.

12

Beyond the Mat

Bridging Yoga and Daily Life

As we embark on this fresh chapter, it's vital to remember that the yoga journey doesn't stop at the edge of your mat. The real magic begins when we seamlessly weave the principles of yoga into the tapestry of our daily lives. Beyond the mat, there lies a world enriched by the transformative power of self-awareness, presence, and alignment, all products of our yoga practice.

Every breath we take, every decision we make, can be imbued with the mindfulness we cultivate on the mat. As you step off your mat and into your life, you step into a world brimming with opportunities for growth and self-improvement.

Reflection Time

Before we delve deeper, let's take a moment to reflect. Grab a notebook or open a new document on your computer, and contemplate on how you've applied the yoga principles we've discussed so far in your daily life. How often do you remember to breathe mindfully during the day? When was the last time you practiced self-compassion outside of your yoga practice? Answering these questions will give you an insight into your current integration of yoga into your life, a necessary first step to further growth.

Transitioning Yoga into Life's Journey

After this reflection, you'll have a better understanding of your starting point. Now, we'll explore techniques to bridge the gap between your yoga mat and your life. To truly live a yogic life means to carry the balance, inner peace, and resilience nurtured on the mat into every corner of our existence.

From mindful communication to conscious eating and from embodying self-love to maintaining balance, we'll delve into all these realms. This chapter will provide practical tools for manifesting your yoga principles in everyday life, thus taking your journey of self-empowerment to unprecedented heights. Remember, your yoga mat is just the beginning; the real journey unfolds as you step beyond it.

Understanding the Benefits of a Daily Yoga Practice

The Miracle of Daily Practice

Yoga, when practiced daily, enriches your life in multiple ways, nurturing your body, mind, and soul. By weaving yoga into your daily routine, you open the doors to a realm of physical, mental, and emotional benefits.

Physically Grounding

Yoga enhances flexibility, strength, and balance. It boosts cardiovascular health and fosters physical resilience. When yoga becomes part of your everyday life, your capacity to navigate life's physical demands improves considerably.

Mentally Nurturing

Yoga encourages mental peace and clarity. The mindful awareness cultivated on the mat can permeate all areas of your life, reducing stress and enhancing decision-making.

Emotionally Empowering

Yoga offers a safe space to connect with our emotions. Regular practice enhances emotional resilience, enabling us to embrace life's highs and lows with equanimity.

The Metamorphosis of Mark

Remember Mark, the high-achieving corporate professional who found his creative side through yoga? When Mark decided to practice yoga daily, he witnessed an even greater transformation. His creativity wasn't just emerging; it was flourishing. The daily practice reinforced his connection with his creative side, improving his problem-solving skills at work and enhancing his personal life. He began painting and even took up creative writing. This newfound joy seeped into all corners of his life, inspiring not only Mark but those around him.

Your Yoga Journey

Now, it's your turn to reflect. How has regular yoga practice impacted your life? Where do you hope to see further improvement or transformation? Identifying these points will help you tailor your practice and set meaningful goals.

The benefits of daily yoga are profound and far-reaching. It's a holistic practice that enhances every facet of your being, preparing you to lead a harmonious life both on and off the mat.

Tips for Integrating Yoga into Your Daily Life

Demystifying Daily Practice

The thought of incorporating yoga into your daily routine can seem daunting, especially with the hustle and bustle of modern life. Yet, with a few practical tips, you can seamlessly weave yoga into your everyday activities, enjoying its benefits on and off the mat.

Morning Energizer

Begin your day with Sun Salutations, a sequence that wakes up the body, enhances flexibility, and sets a mindful tone for your day. It's like sipping on a cup of sunrise, filling you with warmth and energy for the day ahead.

Mid-day Refresher

Try a few stretches or a simple meditation during your lunch break. This can help clear your mind, release tension from your body, and recharge you for the rest of the day. It's like a mini vacation in the midst of your day!

Evening Wind-down

Incorporate restorative yoga poses or a short guided relaxation into your evening routine. This can help you transition from the activities of the day to a peaceful night's sleep. Consider this as tucking your mind and body into bed.

Practical Tip: Yoga Everywhere

Remember, yoga doesn't have to be limited to your mat. Find opportunities throughout your day to practice mindfulness, whether it's while brushing your teeth, walking your dog, or waiting for your coffee to brew. These moments of mindfulness contribute to your yoga practice as much as the poses do.

Your Yoga Planner

Now, let's translate these tips into action. Design a weekly yoga planner tailored to your routine. Divide each day into morning, mid-day, and evening. Schedule a short yoga session for each part of the day, keeping in mind your energy levels and available time. Add in those mindful moments, too. Remember, it's not about doing it all at once; it's about taking small steps towards a more mindful and yogic lifestyle.

Integrating yoga into your daily life doesn't need to be complicated. With these practical tips and your personalized yoga planner, you can enjoy the benefits of yoga every day, creating harmony and balance within and around you. Remember, every breath and every moment can be an extension of your yoga practice.

How Yoga Can Help You Live a More Fulfilling Life

The Fulfillment Factor

Living a fulfilling life goes beyond external achievements. It's about balance, mindfulness, and self-awareness. Yoga, in its profound wisdom, offers a path to all these aspects, guiding you towards a more satisfying and meaningful existence.

Balance: The Art of Harmonious Living

Yoga is not just about balancing on one foot; it's about achieving equilibrium in all areas of life. Through physical poses and breathwork, yoga fosters a deep sense of harmony within, enabling you to navigate life's ups and downs with grace and resilience.

Mindfulness: The Power of Presence

Yoga cultivates mindfulness, the ability to be fully present in each moment. By teaching you to observe your breath and body sensations, yoga anchors you to the here and now, infusing every moment with depth and richness.

Self-Awareness: The Journey Within

At its core, yoga is a journey of self-discovery. It invites you to delve into the layers of your being, fostering a profound sense of self-awareness. This connection with your true self is the cornerstone of a fulfilling life.

Practical Tip: Mindfulness and Meditation

Try incorporating a daily meditation practice to foster mindfulness. Begin with a few minutes each day, focusing on your breath. With time, extend this practice, observing your thoughts and emotions without judgment. This quiet introspection is like shining a light within, illuminating your path to fulfillment.

Your Fulfillment Journal

Take a moment to reflect on what fulfillment means to you. What brings you joy? What makes you feel alive? Use the following prompts to guide your exploration:

1. What aspects of my life bring me the most fulfillment?
2. How does my yoga practice contribute to my sense of fulfillment?
3. How can I further integrate yoga into my life to enhance my sense of fulfillment?

Through its holistic approach, yoga offers a powerful tool for living a fulfilling life. By promoting balance, mindfulness, and self-awareness, it nurtures your well-being on all levels, leading you towards a life of richness and fulfillment. As you continue your yoga journey, remember, each breath, each pose, and each moment of stillness is a step towards a more fulfilling life.

Applying the Principles of Yoga to Your Daily Life

Yoga is more than a set of postures; it's a philosophy of life, a compass guiding you towards balance, compassion, and inner peace. Incorporating yoga principles into your daily life can significantly enhance your personal growth and cultivate harmony in your surroundings.

The Principles: A Closer Look

Let's delve into some key yoga principles and explore how to weave them into the tapestry of your everyday life.

Ahimsa (Non-violence): This principle invites you to practice kindness towards yourself and others. It could be as simple as nurturing self-care habits or choosing compassionate responses in your interactions.

Satya (Truthfulness): By embracing honesty, you foster authentic relationships and live in alignment with your inner truth. This could mean speaking up for what you believe or being true to your commitments.

Santosha (Contentment): This principle encourages an attitude of gratitude and acceptance of life's ups and downs. Cultivate contentment by acknowledging your blessings daily or by practicing mindfulness.

Practical Tip: Living Yoga Daily

Remember, these principles are not rules but guideposts for a fulfilling life. Here are a few techniques to integrate them into your daily routine:

Start your day with a few minutes of reflection, contemplating how you can live the principles of Ahimsa, Satya, and Santosha.

Be mindful during interactions with others. Pause before reacting, choosing a response in line with the principles of non-violence and truth.

End your day with gratitude. Reflect on your experiences and recognize the learning and growth they provided.

Your Yoga in Life Assessment

Now, let's gauge your current understanding and application of these yoga principles in your life. Use the following self-assessment questions to help identify your strengths and areas of growth:

1. How have I practiced Ahimsa (non-violence) in my interactions today?
2. Was there a moment when I could have been more honest (Satya) with myself or others? How will I approach this situation differently next time?
3. Did I acknowledge and appreciate my blessings (Santosha) today? How can I cultivate a more grateful outlook?

Remember, the journey to integrating yoga principles into your daily life is a personal one and unique to each individual. It's not about perfection, but progress. With each step, you're fostering personal growth, enhancing your well-being, and creating ripples of positivity in your world. And in this journey, the mat is your starting point, and the world, your stage. Happy journeying!

Techniques for Living a More Mindful and Fulfilling Life

The Path to Mindfulness

Our lives often whirl around, caught in the flurry of daily tasks, responsibilities, and commitments. Slowing down to cultivate mindfulness can lead to a deeper sense of fulfillment and joy. It's like a voyage of self-discovery, with yoga and meditation as your navigational tools.

Unveiling Mindfulness Techniques

So, how do we embark on this voyage? Here are a few mindfulness techniques that can help you connect deeply with the present moment, thereby infusing your daily life with tranquility and fulfillment.

Yoga: More than just physical exercise, yoga unifies the body, mind, and spirit. It cultivates awareness of your body and breath, grounding you in the present.

Meditation: Through meditation, you learn to observe your thoughts and emotions without judgment. It's a window into your inner landscape, fostering a sense of peace and clarity.

Practical Tip: Embrace the Techniques

Let's break down how to integrate these practices into your daily routine:

Yoga: Start small. Set aside 15-20 minutes each day for a soothing yoga session. Experiment with uncomplicated asanas like Sukhasana (Easy Pose) for grounding, transitioning into Utkata Konasana (Goddess Pose) for strength, and finally settling into Padmasana (Lotus Pose) for meditation. With consistent practice, these poses can serve as your foundation, providing balance, calm, and focus as you embark on your yoga journey.

Meditation: Try a basic mindfulness meditation. Start with just five minutes a day. Sit comfortably, close your eyes, and focus on your breath. When your mind wanders, gently bring your attention back to your breath.

Remember, consistency is key. These practices are most effective when performed regularly.

Your Mindfulness Journey Begins Here

Let's put theory into practice with a guided mindfulness exercise. You don't need any special equipment — just a quiet, comfortable space. Ready? Let's begin.

Sit comfortably, either on a chair or on the floor. Close your eyes and take a deep breath in, then breathe out slowly.

Allow your breath to return to its natural rhythm. Focus on the sensation of breathing in and out.

You may notice your mind wandering. That's okay. When it happens, gently return your attention to your breath.

Continue this for about five minutes. Notice how your body feels. Are you more relaxed? More aware?

Voila! You just practiced mindfulness meditation. Remember, the goal isn't to empty your mind of thoughts, but to observe them without judgment.

Incorporating mindfulness techniques into your daily life paves the way for a more fulfilling existence. Each breath, each yoga pose, each mindful moment is a step towards tranquility and a deeper connection with your inner self. It's a journey well worth embarking on, and every journey begins with a single step. Why not take that step today?

Practicing Gratitude and Cultivating a Positive Mindset

The Power of Gratitude and Positivity

Do you remember that warm, glowing feeling inside when someone expressed genuine gratitude towards you? Or that spark of joy that ignited in your heart when you genuinely appreciated someone's effort? Imagine harnessing that energy every day. Cultivating gratitude and a positive mindset can drastically enhance your life quality, transforming the way you interact with the world.

Intertwining Yoga and Gratitude

Yoga and gratitude share a beautiful relationship. Each asana, each breath, brings you into a space of mindfulness where gratitude naturally thrives. It's an opportunity to express gratitude for your body, your breath, your very existence. This process creates an internal environment conducive to positivity, further fueling gratitude in a virtuous cycle.

Practical Tips: Harnessing Gratitude and Positivity

Let's dive into techniques for fostering gratitude and a positive mindset.

Gratitude Journal: Each day, jot down three things you're grateful for. They can be as simple as a delicious meal, a compliment, or the sound of birds chirping.

Yoga and Meditation: During your practice, dedicate moments to express gratitude. This could be during Savasana (Corpse Pose), when you have the quiet space to reflect.

Affirmations: Positive affirmations can shape your mindset over time. Begin your day by saying something positive to yourself, like "I am capable," "I am grateful," or "I am enough."

Your Gratitude Journal Template

To get you started on your gratitude journey, here's a simple template for your gratitude journal. You can modify it as per your needs.

Date: _____

1. Today, I am grateful for: _____

    Why? _____

2. Today, I am grateful for: _____

    Why? _____

3. Today, I am grateful for: _____

    Why? _____

A Positive Action I Took Today: _____

A Positive Affirmation For Tomorrow: _____

That's it! A small yet significant start to cultivating a practice of gratitude and positivity. Over time, you'll notice a shift in your outlook, leading to a deeper, more fulfilling life experience.

Remember, the journey towards gratitude and a positive mindset is a personal one, and there's no 'right' way to do it. It's not about denying difficulties or forcing happiness. It's about acknowledging life's complexities, appreciating the good, and understanding that challenges are part of the journey. This path, paved with gratitude and positivity, leads towards a life brimming with fulfillment and joy. So, are you ready to take the first step?

Using Your Inner Light to Make a Positive Impact on the World

Unleashing Your Inner Light

In the universe of yoga, we often speak of the "inner light", the radiant energy within that reflects our true essence. This light, powered by love, compassion, and authenticity, holds transformative potential. When we harness our inner light, we not only illuminate our paths but also brighten the world around us.

Your inner light can manifest in diverse ways - a kind word, a helpful act, or simply your joyful presence. Each moment of positivity, no matter how small, contributes to a more loving and peaceful world.

Practical Tips: Igniting Your Inner Light

How can we stoke this inner light? Here are some suggestions:

Daily Meditation: Consistent meditation can help you connect deeper with your inner self, helping your inner light to shine brighter.

For instance, I noticed how a regular 15-minute morning meditation improved my focus throughout the day. More importantly, it helped me handle stress better, making me more patient and present in my interactions with others.

Acts of Kindness: Small gestures of kindness to others can amplify your inner light, creating ripples of positivity.

I recall a time when I helped an elderly lady with her groceries. Her face lit up with gratitude, which in turn filled me with a sense of joy and fulfillment that lasted the entire day. Such simple acts of kindness can indeed make a significant positive impact.

Nurturing Positive Thoughts: Cultivate a habit of positive thinking. This will naturally radiate outward, influencing those around you.

I remember facing a particularly challenging work situation. Rather than allowing myself to be overwhelmed by negativity, I chose to focus on the potential for growth and learning. By maintaining this positive mindset, I was able to navigate the situation more effectively, which also had a calming effect on my team.

Channeling Your Inner Light

Consider these reflective questions:

1. What are some qualities or talents you possess that make you feel genuinely happy and fulfilled?
2. How can you utilize these qualities or talents to make a positive impact on others?
3. Can you recall a time when your actions positively influenced someone's day? How did that make you feel?

Unleashing your inner light isn't about monumental changes but small, consistent actions. By being true to yourself and spreading positivity, you'll inspire others to do the same, lighting up the world one action at a time. The collective radiance of our inner lights has the power to create a global ripple of positivity. So let's ignite our inner light, shall we?

30-Day Yoga Challenge: A Step-by-Step Plan to Integrate Yoga into Your Daily Life

Embarking on a Yoga Journey

Imagine you could seamlessly integrate yoga into your daily life, gaining all its benefits - flexibility, balance, tranquility, and an elevated sense of self-awareness. Our 30-Day Yoga Challenge is the perfect way to jump-start your yoga practice, even amidst a bustling lifestyle.

The beauty of this challenge is its adaptability. Whether you're an early riser or a night owl, a seasoned yogi or a beginner, this plan accommodates everyone. You'll soon find that yoga is less about perfecting asanas and more about deepening your connection with yourself.

Practical Tips: 30 Days of Yoga Bliss

Day 1-7: Introduction and Foundation Building

I remember the first week I started my yoga journey. Despite my enthusiasm, I struggled with even the simplest of poses, feeling awkward and inflexible. It was disheartening at first, but by day 7, I started to notice a slight ease in my movements and a better understanding of my body. This small victory was the push I needed to keep going.

For the first week, focus on getting into the rhythm of daily practice. Start with gentle stretches and foundational poses like Mountain Pose, Child's Pose, Downward Dog, and Warrior I and II. Dedicate at least 15 minutes each day to practice.

Day 8-14: Building Strength and Flexibility

The second week involves adding more strength and flexibility poses. Incorporate poses like Tree Pose, Triangle Pose, and Bridge Pose. Also, try holding poses for a little longer to increase strength and flexibility. Continue with 15-20 minutes daily practice.

Day 15-21: Deepening Your Practice

By now, you'll start to notice changes - a more toned body, a calmer mind, and enhanced flexibility. Now is the time to deepen your practice. Introduce meditation at the beginning or end of your practice. Try new poses like Crow Pose or Camel Pose. Maintain a 20-30 minute practice.

Day 22-30: Cultivating a Personal Practice

By the last week, my journey had transformed from a mere challenge to an essential part of my daily routine. One morning, as I flowed through my Sun Salutations, I realized my body moved with a fluidity and awareness I had never felt before. This realization was a pivotal moment, signifying the birth of my personal yoga practice.

In the final phase, focus on personalizing your practice. Choose poses that resonate with you and help you feel centered. Experiment with sequences that help you flow naturally from one pose to another. Continue your meditation practice and aim for a 30-minute daily session.

Tracking Your Progress

In order to maintain momentum and document your progress throughout the 30-day challenge, we've curated a template for a challenge calendar. You can create your own personalized version using accessible software like Google Sheets or free design platforms like Canva. Once you have your calendar, position it in a noticeable spot, marking each day as you finish your practice. This tangible manifestation of your dedication will bolster your motivation, encouraging you to persist in your transformative journey.

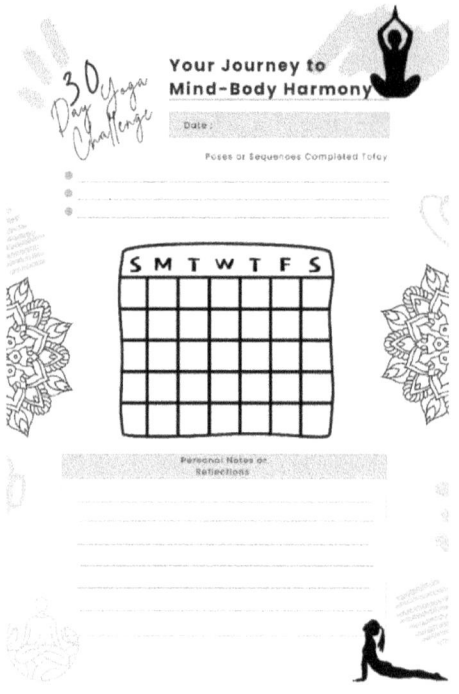

Remember, the aim of this challenge is not perfection, but consistency. It's about showing up for yourself, every single day. By the end of these 30 days, you'll have cultivated a daily yoga habit, reaping its physical, mental, and emotional benefits. So, are you ready to rise to the challenge and welcome yoga into your daily life?

Now that you have completed the 30-Day Yoga Challenge, you have a strong foundation in yoga and a better understanding of your capabilities and preferences. You may have found certain poses more enjoyable or beneficial than others, and you might be wondering what's next. That's where designing your personal yoga practice comes in. This exercise helps you create a yoga routine that is tailored to your unique needs and preferences, ensuring that your yoga practice continues to be a source of joy and fulfillment beyond the 30 days.

Interactive Exercise: Designing Your Personal Yoga Practice

To fully reap the benefits of yoga, it's important to design a practice that resonates with your unique needs, preferences, and lifestyle. Here are some tips to guide you through this process.

Know Your Intent

Before you start designing your yoga practice, you must understand your intent. Are you looking to relieve stress, improve flexibility, build strength, or find a deeper spiritual connection? Your intent will drive the choices you make in your practice.

Assess Your Level and Preferences

Assess your current skill level in yoga – are you a beginner, intermediate, or advanced practitioner? Also, consider the type of yoga that you prefer. Some people enjoy the gentle flow of Hatha yoga, while others prefer the challenging poses of Ashtanga yoga.

Create Your Yoga Sequence

Based on your intent, level, and preferences, you can then create your yoga sequence. A well-rounded sequence should typically include a warm-up, a peak pose, cool-down poses, and a final relaxation pose. If you're unsure, there are plenty of resources online, or you could consult with a yoga instructor.

Plan for Consistency

Finally, determine the frequency and length of your yoga sessions. Consistency is key in yoga, so make sure your schedule is realistic and fits into your daily routine.

Designing Your Personal Yoga Practice Worksheet

Imagine a printable worksheet divided into sections corresponding to the steps above. There would be areas for you to write down your intentions, your level and preferences, your chosen yoga sequence, and your proposed schedule.

Your Intent: Space to write down your goals for your yoga practice.

Your Level and Preferences: Space to note down your skill level and preferred types of yoga.

Your Yoga Sequence: Space to write down your chosen poses, keeping in mind the structure of a typical yoga sequence.

Your Schedule: A table or chart to mark down when and how long you'll practice each day.

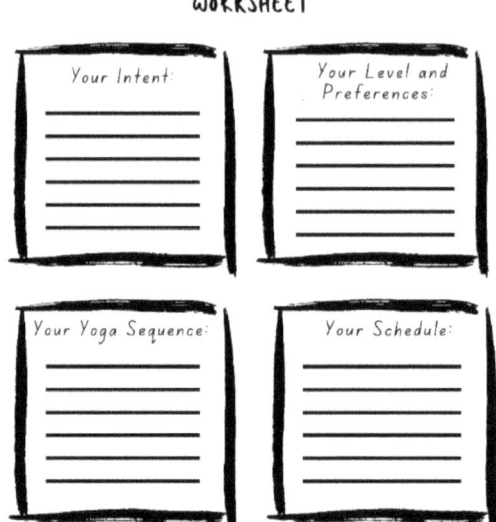

By filling out this worksheet, you will have a clear and personalized roadmap for your yoga journey, setting you up for success.

The Power of Yoga Beyond the Mat

As we wrap up this enlightening journey through yoga, it's important to reflect on the transformative power that this ancient practice holds. Yoga isn't confined to the mat; it's a philosophy, a way of life that transcends the physical realm. When we apply the principles of yoga to our everyday lives, we experience growth in awareness, mindfulness, and tranquility. It brings balance to our body, mind, and spirit, leading to a life of harmony.

So, what's the magic of yoga? It's the power to guide us in times of turbulence, to illuminate our path with inner light, and to awaken gratitude and positivity within us. It's the strength to be found in a simple breath, the joy in a shared smile during a class, or the peace attained through meditation.

Reflect on your journey thus far. How have the principles of yoga touched your life? What changes have you noticed in your mindset, relationships, and overall wellbeing?

As we close this chapter, I challenge you to commit to your yoga practice, to nurture your inner light, and to make an impact on the world around you. Start with one small step—maybe it's a daily gratitude journal or a simple sun salutation every morning. And remember, yoga is not about perfection, but about progress, growth, and self-discovery.

Looking ahead, our next chapter delves into overcoming obstacles on your yoga adventure. It's a journey that requires resilience, a growth mindset, and an embracing of change—skills you've begun to cultivate right here. I'm thrilled to guide you further on this path of transformation and fulfillment.

Remember, yoga is not a destination but a path, a continuous journey of growth and discovery. Let's continue to walk this path together, illuminating our lives with the profound wisdom and transformative power of yoga.

13

Overcoming Obstacles on Your Yoga Adventure

In our yoga journey, the path is not always lit with clarity, sometimes it is dotted with obstacles and challenges. But remember, yoga is not about the absence of problems; it's about using the principles we've learned to overcome them. That's the essence of our discussion in this chapter.

Embracing the Art of Resilience

Each roadblock we face in our yoga journey is an opportunity for growth and self-discovery. This is where resilience plays a vital role. Just as a tree sways in the wind but does not break, we too can learn to sway with life's trials, bending but not breaking. A growth mindset, viewing challenges as catalysts for progress, is paramount in this journey. It pushes us to strive for continuous development, setting a deeper foundation for our yoga practice.

Recognizing the Obstacles

It's essential to acknowledge the hurdles that you might encounter on your path. They could be physical limitations, emotional burdens, lack of time, or even mental blocks. Understanding and identifying these obstacles is the first step in effectively overcoming them. Once recognized, they lose their power to hold us back and become stepping stones, leading us towards a more profound practice.

Discovering Your Challenges

Take a moment now for a bit of self-discovery. Here is a self-assessment quiz to help you identify personal obstacles in your yoga journey. Answer with complete honesty and openness. Remember, there's no judgment here—just an opportunity for introspection and self-improvement. This process will shed light on the areas that may require more attention and serve as a guide to direct your yoga practice more effectively.

As we delve deeper into this chapter, we'll explore how we can employ the transformative power of yoga to face these obstacles head-on. Remember, every obstacle is an opportunity for growth, and every moment of growth brings us closer to our authentic selves. The journey may be challenging, but it is definitely rewarding. Let's embrace it with open arms!

Identifying Common Obstacles in Your Yoga Journey

Common Obstacles in the Yoga Journey

Yoga is a journey of self-discovery, but it's not always a straightforward path. Sometimes, it winds, bends, and throws up obstacles in our way. Some of the common ones that most of us grapple with include a lack of time, physical limitations, and mental blocks.

Time Constraints: The demands of modern life can be relentless, and carving out time for yoga can feel like an insurmountable challenge. But remember, yoga is not just an activity; it's a lifestyle. Even a few moments of mindful breathing in your daily routine can make a world of difference.

Physical Limitations: Not everyone can twist into pretzel-like poses or balance on one foot for minutes at a stretch. But yoga is not just about the asanas (poses). It's about unity—integrating the body, mind, and spirit in harmony.

Mental Blocks: Sometimes, our own minds can be our biggest adversaries, clouded by doubts, fears, and negative self-talk. Overcoming these mental barriers requires patience and compassion towards ourselves.

Personal Story: Overcoming Obstacles

Let's revisit Mark's story here. Mark was a high-achieving corporate professional who began practicing yoga to manage his stress. But he faced an obstacle: he believed he didn't have a 'creative bone' in his body, making certain elements of his yoga practice, like visualization and meditation, challenging. Over time, however, Mark discovered his creative side was not only present but flourishing. He began painting, even took up creative writing. Mark overcame his mental block by embracing the possibility of growth and change in his yoga journey.

Reflecting on Your Journey

Now, it's time for some self-reflection. Take a few moments to consider the obstacles you've faced or are currently facing in your yoga journey. Are you battling time constraints? Are there physical limitations you're trying to work around? Or are mental blocks inhibiting your progress? Recognize these hurdles, just as Mark did, as opportunities for growth. Consider how they can be reshaped into stepping stones toward a deeper, more fulfilling yoga journey.

Remember, the path of yoga, like life, isn't always smooth, but each challenge is an invitation to grow stronger, more resilient, and more self-aware. So, embrace these obstacles, for they are part of your unique yoga adventure.

Strategies for Overcoming Obstacles and Building Resilience

Overcoming Obstacles: Practical Strategies

In the journey of yoga, obstacles are not roadblocks, but signposts for growth and transformation. Here are some strategies that can guide you through:

Plan and Prioritize: If time is your obstacle, consider integrating yoga into your daily routine. Ten minutes of mindful breathing or gentle stretching in the morning can be a great start. Remember, consistency trumps duration.

Adapt and Modify: Physical limitation is an obstacle that can be worked around by adapting postures to your own body. Yoga is not a competition; it's a personal journey. Always honor your body's unique needs and capabilities.

Cultivate Mindfulness: For mental blocks, mindfulness can be your key. Whether it's through meditation or mindful yoga practice, allow yourself to observe your thoughts and emotions without judgment. Over time, this awareness can help dismantle these blocks.

Building Resilience: A Journey, Not a Destination

Resilience is like a muscle, the more you use it, the stronger it gets. And yoga provides the perfect playground for developing this muscle. Whether it's holding a challenging pose for a few more breaths, or practicing detachment in the face of a wandering mind during meditation, each moment in yoga teaches us resilience.

Practical Tip: Embracing Change

Change is a part of life, but it's often a cause for stress. A technique to practice resilience in the face of change is to embrace it as an opportunity for growth. On your yoga mat, this might mean trying a new pose or a different style of yoga. Off the mat, it could translate to welcoming a new project at work or adapting to a shift in your personal life with an open, receptive mind.

Resilience-Building Exercise

Now, let's practice this resilience-building exercise together. Find a comfortable seated position. Close your eyes and take a few deep breaths. Now, visualize an obstacle you're currently facing in your yoga journey. It could be a challenging pose, a mental block, or a scheduling conflict.

Once you have this obstacle in mind, ask yourself: What is one small step I can take today to navigate this obstacle? It might be waking up 10 minutes earlier for a brief morning practice, or seeking guidance from a yoga teacher for a difficult pose, or writing down your thoughts and feelings to better understand your mental block.

Open your eyes. Jot down this step in your yoga journal and commit to practicing it. This simple exercise is an act of resilience, a commitment to overcoming an obstacle, one step at a time.

Remember, resilience isn't about never facing difficulties; it's about navigating them with grace and determination. And every time you step onto your yoga mat, you're building this resilience, strengthening your ability to overcome obstacles on your yoga adventure. So, keep practicing, keep growing, and keep shining!

Developing a Growth Mindset through Yoga

Understanding Growth Mindset

A "growth mindset" refers to the belief that our abilities and intelligence can be developed through dedication and hard work. This perspective fosters a love for learning, the courage to face challenges, and the resilience to recover from setbacks. Contrastingly, a "fixed mindset" holds the view that our capabilities are innate and unchangeable.

In the context of yoga, a growth mindset can manifest as the willingness to explore new asanas (postures), the openness to delve into yoga philosophy, or the resolve to maintain a consistent practice, even when progress seems slow.

Cultivating Growth Mindset Through Yoga

Yoga is a fantastic tool to nurture a growth mindset. It's not just about bending our bodies into poses, but also about flexing our minds, transforming our thoughts, and expanding our understanding of ourselves.

Embrace the Beginner's Mind: In yoga, having a 'beginner's mind' means approaching your practice with curiosity and openness, no matter your level of experience. This perspective aligns perfectly with a growth mindset and encourages continual learning.

Practice Non-Judgment: Yoga teaches us to be present and accept each moment as it is. This attitude of non-judgment can extend to our perception of our abilities, facilitating a shift from a fixed mindset to a growth mindset.

Celebrate Small Victories: In yoga, every effort is meaningful, whether it's holding a pose for a second longer or finding a deeper level of relaxation in savasana. Recognizing and celebrating these moments can foster a growth mindset, focusing on progress rather than perfection.

Practical Tip: The Mind-Body Connection

One technique to nurture a growth mindset through yoga is to consciously connect with your body during your practice. As you move into a pose, instead of striving for a perfect shape, try to tune into the sensations in your body, observe your breath, and notice your thoughts. This mindful attention encourages a deeper connection with your inner self, fostering an understanding that growth is an inward journey of self-discovery and self-improvement.

Guided Meditation for Growth Mindset

Let's put these concepts into practice with a guided meditation. Find a quiet, comfortable space and sit with your spine tall and your eyes gently closed.

Take a few deep, grounding breaths, then allow your breath to settle into its natural rhythm. Imagine yourself standing at the base of a mountain, your mountain of growth. As you look up at this mountain, recognize that it symbolizes your potential for growth and learning.

With each breath in, feel your courage grow, your determination solidify. With each breath out, let go of doubts, of fear. Now, begin your ascent. Each step up this mountain symbolizes progress, however small. Sometimes, the path may seem steep, but remind yourself: progress, not perfection.

As you reach the summit, allow yourself a moment to celebrate this journey of growth. When you're ready, slowly open your eyes, carrying this growth mindset into your yoga practice and your daily life.

Remember, growth isn't always linear, and setbacks are part of the process. But with a growth mindset nurtured through yoga, you're equipped with the resilience and open-mindedness to continue your unique journey of self-discovery and transformation.

Customizing Your Yoga Practice to Suit Your Lifestyle and Needs

Personalizing Your Yoga Journey

Yoga is a personal journey, and what works for one individual might not work for another. As we progress on this path, it becomes essential to adapt our yoga practice to our unique lifestyle, needs, and even limitations. Remember, yoga is not about conforming to an ideal—it's about tuning into our bodies and honoring our individual journey.

Adapting Yoga to Your Lifestyle and Needs

Personalizing your yoga practice means understanding your physical needs, emotional state, and schedule constraints.

Listen to Your Body: Your body is your most reliable guide. If certain poses don't feel right, adapt them or replace them with others that serve you better. Props can also be valuable tools for accommodating physical limitations or injuries.

Align with Your Emotional State: Your emotional state significantly influences your practice. If you're feeling energetic, a vigorous vinyasa flow might suit you. On stressful days, restorative yoga or a calming meditation can be more beneficial.

Respect Your Schedule: We all lead busy lives, and it's important to incorporate yoga in a way that complements your lifestyle. Perhaps a morning routine energizes you for the day, or an evening practice helps you unwind. Even a short 15-minute practice can make a significant impact when done consistently.

Practical Tip: Customizing Your Yoga Routine

When designing your routine, focus on creating a balanced practice. Start with a warm-up to prepare your body, move into more challenging asanas, and end with a cooldown to ground and relax your body. Don't forget to incorporate pranayama (breathing techniques) and meditation for a holistic practice.

Your Personal Yoga Practice Worksheet

Let's put these principles into practice with a worksheet designed to help you create your customized yoga routine.

1. **Daily Schedule**

    - Time of day for practice: _____

    - Duration of practice: _____

2. **Physical Needs**

    - Areas of the body to focus on: _____

    - Any limitations to consider: _____

3. **Emotional State**

    - Current emotional state: _____

    - Desired emotional state post-practice: _____

4. **Yoga Routine**

    - Warm-up poses: _____

    - Main practice poses: _____

    - Cool down poses: _____

    - Pranayama techniques: _____

    - Meditation practice: _____

Feel free to revisit this worksheet as often as needed, adapting it as you evolve in your yoga journey. By customizing your practice, you'll cultivate a deeper connection with yourself, making your yoga journey a truly personal adventure of growth and transformation.

Navigating Plateaus and Stagnation in Your Yoga Practice

Understanding Plateaus and Stagnation

In your yoga journey, you may encounter periods of stagnation or plateaus - times when you feel stuck, no longer progressing, or even regressing. Such times can be disheartening, making you question the value of your practice. However, it's essential to realize that these plateaus are a normal part of any growth process, including yoga.

Why Do Plateaus Happen?

Plateaus can result from various factors, such as repetitiveness, loss of focus, or physical or mental exhaustion. They may also signal that your body and mind are ready for a new challenge or a different approach.

Practical Tip: Overcoming Stagnation

The key to breaking through a plateau is reigniting your passion, challenging yourself, and bringing mindfulness back into your practice.

Embrace Variety: Mixing up your yoga routine can help stimulate growth. Try new poses, explore different yoga styles, or incorporate a new pranayama or meditation technique.

Set New Goals: If your practice has become too comfortable, it might be time to set a new challenge. This could be mastering a complex pose, deepening your meditation practice, or refining your alignment in certain asanas.

Mindful Practice: Bring fresh attention to your practice. Focus on the sensations in each pose, the rhythm of your breath, and the state of your mind. This mindfulness can bring new depth to your practice.

Identifying and Overcoming Plateaus

Here are some reflection questions to help you identify any plateaus and brainstorm ways to overcome them:

1. Have you noticed any stagnation or lack of progress in your yoga practice recently? In what ways?

2. What might be causing this plateau? (Consider aspects such as repetitiveness, lack of focus, exhaustion, etc.)

3. What new elements can you introduce to your practice to break through this plateau? (Consider variety, new goals, mindfulness, etc.)

4. How do you feel about these changes? Are there any potential challenges, and how can you address them?

Remember, plateaus aren't a failure but a call for transformation. By acknowledging them and proactively seeking to overcome them, you can turn these perceived obstacles into powerful catalysts for growth and deeper understanding in your yoga journey.

Embracing Change and Transformation on Your Yoga Path

The Impermanence of Life and Yoga

The only constant in life is change. Just as the seasons change, so do we - mentally, physically, emotionally. In yoga, this continuous evolution is at the heart of the journey. Each pose, each breath, each moment of mindfulness is an opportunity for transformation.

Accepting Change

Resisting change can lead to stress and suffering. Embracing it, however, cultivates resilience and opens us up to personal growth. Yoga teaches us to accept change - to flow with it, rather than against it.

Practical Tip: Mindfulness for Change

A powerful tool to help you embrace change is mindfulness. By staying present in each moment, you learn to accept things as they are, without clinging to how they were or how you want them to be. Here's a simple mindfulness practice:

1. Start in a comfortable seated position.
2. Bring your awareness to your breath, noticing its natural rhythm.
3. When your mind wanders, gently bring it back to your breath.
4. As thoughts or feelings about change arise, acknowledge them without judgement and let them go, bringing your focus back to your breath.
5. Practice this for a few minutes daily.

Guided Visualization

Now, let's try a guided visualization to help embrace change and transformation. Close your eyes and visualize yourself standing beside a calm, flowing river.

1. Imagine this river represents your life's journey, constantly changing, flowing.
2. See yourself stepping into the river, feel the cool water, notice it moving around you.

3. Visualize how the river adapts to you stepping into it - changing course, moving around you, but always continuing to flow.
4. Acknowledge this as a symbol of life's changes. Notice any resistance and let it go. Embrace the flow of change.

Through yoga, you can develop the ability to flow with life's transformations. As you continue your practice, remember that change is a vital part of your journey. Embrace it with an open heart and mind, and let it guide you towards growth and self-discovery.

Identifying and Overcoming Your Personal Obstacles

Recognizing Your Hurdles

The first step in any journey of growth is acknowledging where you're starting. In your yoga practice, identifying personal obstacles can illuminate your path to progress. Are you struggling with consistency? Do you find certain poses challenging? Or maybe your challenge is mental – anxiety, self-doubt, or lack of focus.

Practical Tip: Conquering Obstacles

Follow these steps to face your obstacles head-on:

Reflect: Identify the biggest obstacles in your yoga practice. They could be physical, mental, or circumstantial.

Analyze: Understand why these are obstacles for you. Are they related to time management, physical capability, or mental blocks?

Plan: Design a strategy to tackle these obstacles. For physical hurdles, consider incorporating specific asanas or exercises into your routine. For mental blocks, meditation or breathing exercises might help.

Execute: Put your plan into action and observe how it works.

Revise: If needed, adjust your strategy based on your observations.

Obstacle Identification and Overcoming Worksheet

Now, it's time to put this into practice. Here's a simple worksheet layout to guide you:

Obstacle Identification: List the top three obstacles you're facing in your yoga journey.

Obstacle Analysis: Write down why each of these is an obstacle for you.

Action Plan: For each obstacle, devise a practical strategy to overcome it.

Reflection: After a week or two of implementing your action plan, note any progress or changes you've observed.

Remember, progress isn't linear. Overcoming obstacles takes patience and resilience. Celebrate your small victories, and view any setbacks as opportunities to learn and grow. Keep refining your strategy as you continue on your journey, embracing the transformations that come with overcoming obstacles.

Guided Meditation: Overcoming Obstacles and Embracing Growth

Creating Your Meditation Space

Before we delve into the guided meditation, let's establish a conducive environment. Clean and declutter your meditation space. Choose a spot where you can be free from interruptions. Dim the lights or light a candle, and consider adding calming scents like lavender or chamomile. This setting will facilitate a peaceful, immersive meditation experience.

Practical Tip: Always remember, consistency is key in meditation. Choose a time of day when you're least likely to be disturbed and commit to it daily.

Guided Meditation: Overcoming Obstacles

1. Sit comfortably, close your eyes and take a few deep breaths.
2. Envision a mountain, symbolic of your personal obstacles.
3. As you inhale, visualize a glowing light in your heart center, representing your inner strength.
4. On each exhale, imagine the light chipping away at the mountain.
5. Continue this visualization, observing as the mountain slowly erodes, making way for a clear path.

6. Open your eyes gently, carrying this visualization into your waking life.

By visualizing your obstacles as a mountain and your resilience as a powerful light, you're programming your subconscious mind to tackle any hurdles with strength and perseverance.

Inspiring Stories of Yoga Transformations

Stories of Resilience and Transformation

Yoga is not only a physical practice but also a transformative journey, and personal obstacles are part of that journey. Let's delve into some inspiring stories from individuals who overcame obstacles and experienced transformations through yoga.

From High-Achieving Professional to Creative Force: Revisiting Mark's Story

We met Mark earlier and revisited him in Chapter 13. A high-achieving corporate professional, he started his yoga journey to manage stress. His biggest obstacle? Believing he lacked creativity, making visualization and meditation challenging. But through consistent yoga practice, Mark embraced change and discovered a flourishing creative side.

Mark started painting and ventured into creative writing. His life transformed as his inner shine emerged, touching his professional work and personal life alike. This newfound joy was infectious, inspiring not only Mark but also those around him.

From Overwhelmed Lawyer to Fulfilled Educator: David's Journey

David, a successful lawyer, often felt overwhelmed despite his professional achievements. Seeking balance, he took up yoga and meditation. Through this journey, he realized his underlying passion for teaching.

David made a bold move - transitioning from his legal career to education. It was challenging, but yoga's teachings of acceptance and resilience guided him. Today, David finds immense satisfaction and happiness in nurturing young minds.

Embracing Change: The Story of Lisa, the Violinist

Remember Lisa? An incredibly skilled violinist, she had kept her talent hidden for years. However, yoga helped her realize the significance of her gift, sparking a life-altering decision.

She transitioned from her regular job to becoming a professional violinist. This leap of faith brought fulfillment to her life and joy to her audience. She overcame her fear and embraced the power of change, all thanks to her yoga journey.

Practical Tip: Overcoming Your Personal Obstacles

What can we learn from these stories? Each individual faced personal obstacles, but yoga offered them a path to navigate through. Remember, the yoga mat is a reflection of life. If you can breathe, balance, and flow through a challenging pose, you can apply the same principles to life's challenges. Your yoga journey is your personal story of transformation - embrace it, for every obstacle overcome is a step towards growth.

The Power of Overcoming Obstacles

Embracing the challenge of personal obstacles is a profound and empowering part of your yoga journey. Each time you encounter an obstacle and overcome it, you are not only growing but also unlocking an inner power that helps you rise above any future challenges.

Embrace the Transformation

From Mark's discovery of his creative side to David's transition into a career of fulfillment, we have witnessed firsthand the transformative power of facing and overcoming obstacles. Remember, yoga isn't just about getting into a pose. It's about the journey - the learning, growing, and transforming - that comes with each breath and movement.

Your Action Plan: Charting the Course Ahead

Now it's your turn. It's time to outline your plans for overcoming your personal obstacles in your yoga journey. Here is an interactive action plan template:

Identify Your Obstacle: What personal obstacle do you currently face in your yoga practice?

Develop a Strategy: What steps can you take to overcome this obstacle?

Set a Timeline: When will you begin implementing this strategy? When do you hope to overcome this obstacle?

Identify Support: Who or what can support you as you work to overcome this obstacle?

Celebrate Progress: How will you celebrate each small step forward?

Remember, the power to overcome obstacles lies within you, and your yoga practice is a tool to unlock that power.

As we conclude this chapter, reflect on the stories of transformation we've discussed. How do these resonate with your journey? Are there techniques or approaches that you're excited to try? What does the power of overcoming obstacles mean to you?

Let's keep the momentum going as we move into the next chapter, where we'll explore how to cultivate compassion through yoga. In Chapter 14, we'll delve into heart-opening poses, techniques for developing self-compassion, and ways to foster compassion in our relationships and community. Get ready to unlock the transformative power of compassion in your yoga journey!

14

Cultivating Compassion through Yoga

Opening the Heart to Compassion

As we turn a new page, we shift our focus from overcoming obstacles to embracing one of the most transformative elements in yoga – compassion. Like a blooming lotus in the pond of our hearts, compassion is an innate part of our being, waiting to be nurtured. In yoga, it's not just about the asanas, it's about the emotional transformation that we nurture within ourselves, one of which is compassion.

The Power of Compassion in Yoga

When we speak of compassion in yoga, we don't only refer to self-compassion but also to our relationships with others. It's about finding a balance between nurturing self-love and spreading that love outwards to those around us. Yoga teaches us that all beings are interconnected. As we foster compassion, we're not only growing personally, but we're also strengthening our social relationships, creating a ripple effect of positivity.

Compassion Self-Assessment

Before diving into techniques and poses for cultivating compassion, it's essential to understand your current capacity for compassion. This self-assessment will help to illuminate where you're starting from, and guide your progression as you move forward:

1. **Compassion Towards Self:** How often do you practice self-love and self-forgiveness?

2. **Compassion Towards Others:** How readily do you empathize with and support others?
3. **Interconnectedness:** Do you recognize and value the interconnectedness of all beings?

Score yourself on a scale of 1-10 for each area. The aim is not to judge, but to recognize where you stand and identify areas for growth. This self-awareness is the first step in cultivating compassion through yoga.

Throughout this chapter, we'll explore heart-opening poses, delve into practices for self-compassion, and learn to extend this compassion to our community. It's a journey of nurturing our capacity to love and be loved - the very essence of yoga. Welcome to this transformative journey of compassion.

Understanding the Importance of Compassion

Compassion: The Heart of Yoga

Yoga transcends physical movement; it's an emotional journey, a spiritual transformation. At its core lies compassion, a subtle, yet profound element, one that affects our mental health and well-being. This universal quality of empathy and understanding doesn't merely pertain to our relationship with others. It begins within us, as self-compassion.

Cultivating compassion through yoga teaches us to be gentle with ourselves, to acknowledge our limitations and imperfections, and to extend this understanding towards others. It has a ripple effect on our mental health, reducing stress and anxiety, enhancing emotional resilience, and fostering a deep sense of interconnectedness. Compassion in yoga is not a destination, but an ongoing journey towards personal growth and meaningful relationships.

Compassion in Action: Mark's Journey Continued

As an extension of Mark's journey we touched upon in Chapter 13, let's examine how compassion played a pivotal role in his transformation. When Mark discovered his creative side, it wasn't a sudden epiphany. It was the result of compassion towards himself - recognizing his fears, acknowledging his challenges, and allowing himself the space to explore and grow without judgment.

Mark started embracing the fluctuations in his yoga journey, instead of resisting them. His practice became less about perfection and more about patience, less about achievement and more about acceptance. His newfound compassion didn't just fuel his creativity but improved his mental health, fostered deeper connections, and enhanced his overall well-being.

Cultivating Compassion in Your Life

Reflection is a powerful tool to nurture compassion. Consider these questions to identify areas where you can cultivate more compassion:

1. How do you treat yourself when you fail or make a mistake?
2. How patient are you with your own growth and progress?
3. How empathetic and understanding are you towards others' struggles and challenges?

Identifying your responses will illuminate areas where you can cultivate compassion. Whether it's being kinder to yourself, or extending empathy to others, every step towards compassion counts.

As we delve further into this chapter, remember that compassion, like yoga, is a practice. It is a journey of discovery, of openness, and of growth - and it begins within you. Let's continue to unlock the transformative power of compassion in our yoga journey.

Yoga Poses and Practices to Open the Heart

Opening the Heart with Yoga

The heart - the center of our emotions, compassion, and connection. Yoga is a wonderful way to unlock this powerful space within us, fostering empathy and compassion. Let's delve into yoga poses and practices that specifically target the heart, helping us radiate love from within.

Pose 1: Supported Fish Pose (Salamba Matsyasana)

To begin, Supported Fish Pose invites openness in the heart and thoracic spine. It encourages deep breaths, nourishing the body with positivity and releasing stress.

To practice, place a bolster or two blocks behind you, at about mid-back, one higher for your head. Sit in front of the bolster and slowly recline back onto it. Keep your legs extended or folded in Sukhasana (Easy Pose). Let your arms rest on the floor, palms up. Breathe deeply and stay for 1-2 minutes.

Pose 2: Wild Thing (Camatkarasana)

Wild Thing is a dynamic heart opener that strengthens and stretches the entire body. This pose represents the joy of living and love for oneself.

Start in Downward-Facing Dog. Extend your right leg back and bend the knee, bringing the heel towards the glutes. Open your hips to the right. Slowly flip your dog, landing softly on your right foot. Extend the right arm forward. Remember to breath deeply, feeling the heart opening with each breath. Hold for 3-5 breaths and repeat on the other side.

Practical Tip: A Gentle Reminder

Remember, the journey of yoga isn't about touching your toes; it's about what you discover along the way. Keep patience and compassion towards yourself as you explore these poses. They should create space, not strain. Modify as needed, using props like blocks and bolsters to support your practice.

A Heart-Opening Yoga Sequence

A short Hatha Yoga Practice for Heart Opening

Welcome to this short heart-opening yoga sequence that encourages compassion and inner connection. Listen to your body and modify as needed. Take as many breaths in each pose that feels right to you, although try not to cheat yourself and hold each pose for a minimum of 3 to 5 breaths. Let's begin!

1. Savasana (Corpse Pose)
   - Lie on your back on your mat with your arms relaxed at your sides, palms facing upwards.
   - Take deep breaths, inviting peace and tranquility.

[Modification: For lower back comfort, place a bolster under your knees.]

2. Warm-up with Cat-Cow Pose

- Come to all fours on your mat. Ensure your wrists are aligned under your shoulders and your knees under your hips.
- As you inhale, lift your chest and tailbone towards the ceiling, letting your belly sink towards the floor (Cow Pose).
- On the exhale, round your spine up towards the ceiling, tucking your chin to your chest (Cat Pose).
- Continue to move between Cow and Cat on the breath for 1-2 minutes, focusing on the heart space as you move.

[Modification: If your wrists hurt, you can make fists or use yoga blocks under your hands.]

3. Supported Fish Pose (Salamba Matsyasana)
   - Position a bolster or two blocks behind you, one at mid-back and one for your head.
   - Sit in front of the bolster, legs extended or folded in Sukhasana (Easy Pose).
   - Lean back onto the bolster and relax, arms open to the side, palms up.

[Modification: Use more or thicker props if your back feels strained.]

4. Gate Pose (Parighasana)
   - Kneel on your mat, extending your right leg to the right.
   - Inhale, raise your left arm, and as you exhale, lean to the right.
   - Hold for 3 breaths, then switch sides.

[Modification: If kneeling is uncomfortable, place a folded blanket under your knees.]

5. Wild Thing (Camatkarasana)
   - Start in Downward-Facing Dog. Lift your right leg back and bend the knee, flipping your dog and landing gently on your right foot.
   - Extend your right arm, opening your heart to the sky.
   - Repeat on the left side.

[Modification: Practice Three-Legged Downward Dog, keeping both hands grounded.]

6. Goddess Pose (Utkata Konasana)

- Stand tall, feet wider than hip-distance apart, toes turned out.
- Bend your knees, lowering your hips into a squat.
- Bring your hands together in prayer position at your heart.

[Modification: Don't squat as deeply if your thighs feel overworked.]

7. Garland Pose (Malasana)
   - Begin in Mountain Pose (Tadasana), then step your feet about mat's width apart.
   - Bend your knees and lower your hips, coming into a squat. Try to keep your heels on the ground. If that's not possible, you can roll up a blanket or mat under your heels for support.
   - Bring your palms together in a prayer position at your chest, and gently press your elbows against the inner knees. This action helps to open the hips even further.
   - Keep your spine long, your chest lifted, and your gaze forward. Hold for 5-7 breaths.

[Modification: If the squat is too intense, you can sit on a block or bolster to elevate the hips.]

8. Lotus Pose (Padmasana)
   - Sit on your mat, bringing your right foot onto your left thigh, then your left foot onto your right thigh.
   - Keep your spine straight and place your hands on your knees, palms up.
   - Close your eyes and take deep breaths, focusing on opening your heart.

[Modification: If full Lotus is uncomfortable, try Half Lotus, placing only one foot on the opposite thigh.]

9. Savasana (Corpse Pose)
   - Lie back on your mat, legs falling open, arms at your sides.
   - Relax and breathe deeply, allowing your body to absorb the benefits of the practice.

[Modification: Place a bolster under your knees for added lower back support.]

This sequence offers heart-opening poses to enhance compassion and empathy. Move mindfully, honoring your body and its limits. Close your practice with a few moments of silence in Savasana, acknowledging the open heart and tranquility you've nurtured.

To conclude, slowly rise to a seated position. Bring your hands to heart center, expressing gratitude for your practice.

Namaste.

Remember, your yoga practice is a journey of self-discovery. As you explore these heart-opening poses, be aware of the emotions that arise. Use them as a mirror, reflecting the state of your heart. And as you breathe into each pose, visualize each breath nurturing your heart, filling it with love, compassion, and peace.

Yoga is more than a physical journey. It's an exploration of the inner self, a journey into the heart. As you open your heart through these practices, you open yourself to the endless possibilities of love and compassion.

Embracing the Art of Self-Compassion: Techniques for Developing Self-Compassion

One of the transformative lessons yoga teaches us is the importance of self-compassion. It's the gentle reminder to treat ourselves with the same kindness we would extend to others. Developing self-compassion is a journey, one that we can nurture through yoga, meditation, and mindfulness. It becomes a warm, steady light in our lives, guiding us through challenges with kindness and grace.

Integrating Self-Compassion through Yoga

Yoga is more than a physical practice; it's a spiritual journey, a deep dive into the self. Each pose and breath is an opportunity to connect with our inner selves, to offer grace in the face of imperfection, and to remember that progress is more important than perfection. When we stumble in a pose or find our minds wandering during meditation, self-compassion encourages us to meet these moments with kindness, to tell ourselves, "It's okay."

Mindful Meditation and Self-Compassion

Meditation offers us a quiet space to nurture self-compassion. When we meditate, we give ourselves the gift of time and space, free from judgment or expectation. Begin by focusing on your breath, then allow your thoughts to arise naturally. Meet each thought with understanding and compassion, as if it were a friend sharing a concern. Let go of self-criticism and replace it with self-understanding. The more we practice this during meditation, the easier it becomes to carry self-compassion into our daily lives.

Practicing Self-Compassion in Daily Life

Here are a few practical ways to nurture self-compassion daily:

1. **Speak kindly to yourself:** The way we speak to ourselves matters. Replace critical self-talk with supportive, kind words.
2. **Journaling:** Write down your feelings, acknowledging your struggles and victories. Appreciate yourself for both.
3. **Mindfulness:** Practice being present in the moment, accepting it without judgment.
4. **Interactive Self-Compassion Exercise:** The Compassionate Hand

This is a tangible, powerful way to connect with self-compassion. Find a quiet place, take a few deep breaths, then place your hand over your heart. Feel the warmth, the gentle rhythm. This is you, offering comfort to yourself. Whisper or think of a phrase that resonates with kindness. It could be as simple as "I am enough" or "I am doing my best". Repeat this daily.

Developing self-compassion isn't a one-time event; it's an ongoing practice, a journey of self-discovery. Remember, you deserve your kindness as much as anyone else. As we cultivate self-compassion, we not only find greater peace within ourselves but we also become a beacon of kindness, lighting the way for others on their own self-compassion journey.

Fostering Compassion in Relationships and Community

Cultivating Compassion in Relationships and Community

Self-compassion, as we learned in the previous section, is an essential ingredient to a fulfilling and peaceful life. However, the circle of compassion doesn't end with the self. Its radiating warmth extends to our relationships and the community we dwell in. Let's explore how the compassion fostered through yoga and mindfulness can enrich our connections and contribute to a more empathetic community.

The Ripple Effect: Compassion in Relationships

The gentle embrace of compassion cultivated through yoga touches not just us but everyone around us. When we nurture compassion within, our interactions with others begin to reflect it. We listen more, understand better, and love deeper. Relationships, whether with a partner, a friend, or family, thrive on this nurturing energy. We become more patient, forgiving, and understanding, leading to healthier, more resilient bonds.

Compassionate Communities: Fostering Unity and Understanding

A community infused with compassion becomes a harbor of understanding and support. It's about showing up for each other, whether it's celebrating victories or navigating challenges. As we extend our yoga and mindfulness practice beyond the mat, we influence our community with our kindness and empathy.

Practical Tips: Living Compassionately

Here are a few ways to integrate compassion into your daily interactions and contribute to a compassionate community:

1. **Active Listening:** In conversations, give your undivided attention. This simple act conveys respect and compassion.
2. **Mindful Speech:** Before speaking, pause. Choose words that build rather than break.
3. **Community Service:** Volunteering in your community not only helps others but strengthens your compassion muscles.

Compassion in Action

Reflect on these questions:

1. In what ways can you show more compassion in your relationships?
2. How can you contribute to building a more compassionate community?
3. How has your yoga and mindfulness practice impacted your approach towards others? Have you noticed any changes in your responses or interactions?

The journey of compassion, like yoga, begins within us but doesn't stop there. It reverberates outwards, touching lives, and nurturing connections. As we become more compassionate, we foster a world that's kinder and more understanding. It starts with a single compassionate act, a word, a gesture. So, let's take our yoga practice off the mat and into the world, cultivating a community and relationships anchored in compassion.

Guided Meditation: Cultivating Loving-Kindness (Metta)

The practice of Loving-Kindness, or Metta meditation, is a powerful tool for fostering compassion towards oneself and others. It invites us to soften our hearts and extend unconditional kindness and love.

Creating a Conducive Environment for Meditation

First, it's crucial to find a quiet, comfortable place where you can meditate without disturbance. Feel free to use cushions or blankets for support. Dim the lights if you can, and if you like, light a candle or some incense to create a serene ambiance. The goal is to make your space feel welcoming and safe, a refuge for your practice.

Step-by-Step Guided Loving-Kindness Meditation

1. Begin by finding a comfortable seated position. Close your eyes, and take a few deep breaths, tuning into the rhythm of your breathing.
2. With every exhale, visualize releasing any tension or negative energy. With each inhale, draw in tranquility and peace.

3. Now, focus on your heart center. Visualize a warm, bright light emanating from it, expanding with each breath. This light symbolizes love and kindness.
4. Repeat the following phrases silently to yourself, directing them towards yourself: "May I be safe. May I be healthy. May I be happy. May I live with ease."
5. Once you feel the warmth and kindness directed towards yourself, picture a loved one. Extend these wishes to them: "May you be safe. May you be healthy. May you be happy. May you live with ease."
6. Gradually extend this loving-kindness to others—friends, neutral individuals, even people you find challenging.
7. Finally, visualize this radiant, loving energy expanding outwards from your heart to your community, the world, and all beings.

The beauty of Metta meditation lies in its simplicity. Remember, it's about cultivating an attitude of love and kindness. Some days it may flow easily, other times it might feel harder. Regardless, every time you practice, you're nurturing your capacity for compassion. With regular practice, you'll notice this loving-kindness extending into your daily life, enriching your interactions and relationships.

Interactive Exercise: Compassionate Journaling

In this chapter, we will delve into the world of compassionate journaling, a practice designed to foster empathy and self-compassion. It is a unique technique that focuses on harnessing the power of words to nurture a compassionate spirit.

How to Practice Compassionate Journaling

Unlike traditional journaling, compassionate journaling involves conscious reflection on our feelings, actions, and reactions from a place of kindness. It encourages us to approach our experiences without judgment but with understanding and love.

To begin, find a quiet, comfortable space where you can write without distractions. Create a serene environment – perhaps light a candle or play some soothing music. Most importantly, approach this exercise with an open heart and mind.

Journal Prompts for Compassionate Journaling

1. Reflect on a recent experience where you felt you lacked self-compassion. How could you have responded more kindly to yourself?
2. Write a letter to your younger self. What words of kindness, advice, or reassurance would you share?
3. Think about someone who's recently upset you. Try to understand their perspective and write about what they might have been feeling.
4. Write down an aspect about yourself that you struggle to accept. How can you extend compassion towards this part of yourself?

Remember, compassionate journaling is a practice. The more you engage with it, the more natural it will become. Over time, you'll notice this compassion extending not only to your journal entries but also into your interactions with yourself and others. This practice is about cultivating a heart that's understanding and kind, even when faced with life's many challenges. By showing compassion to ourselves on paper, we learn how to do so in our real-life experiences. It's an exercise in humanity and understanding, as we learn to give ourselves and others the grace we all deserve.

Practicing Yoga for Social Change and Activism

Yoga is more than a personal journey; it's a pathway to societal transformation. Rooted in the principles of ahimsa (non-violence) and compassion, yoga encourages us to see the interconnectedness of all life, inspiring us to act for social change.

Yoga, Compassion, and Social Change

Compassion is a cornerstone of yoga philosophy, inviting us to extend empathy and understanding, first towards ourselves and then towards others. Compassion propels us to take action, to alleviate suffering and injustice wherever we see it. It's the bridge between personal transformation and societal change.

Just as our yoga practices evolve, so does our capacity for compassion. Through mindful movement and conscious breathing, we nurture a sense of interconnectedness and empathy. We realize that our well-being is intertwined with the well-being of our society and our planet. This understanding inspires us to utilize yoga as a tool for social activism.

Personal Story: Yoga and Social Activism

Let's revisit Sarah's story. You remember Sarah, the busy mother who discovered her talent for painting through mindfulness and yoga. With her creative spirit kindled, Sarah began to notice the world around her in new ways. She saw the beauty in everyday life but also the areas of injustice and suffering that needed attention.

Sarah started painting murals in her community, depicting themes of unity, peace, and resilience. Her art became a powerful tool for social activism, sparking conversations about societal issues and bringing her community together. The compassion she cultivated on the yoga mat extended to her creative work and social activism. Her story illustrates the transformational power of yoga - not just for the individual, but for communities and societies.

Reflection: Yoga and Your Contribution to Social Change

Let's consider how you can channel your yoga practice for social change. Reflect on these questions:

1. How has yoga increased your awareness of social issues or injustice?
2. In what ways has your yoga practice nurtured compassion towards yourself and others?
3. How can you use this compassion to effect change within your community or in the wider society?

We each have unique gifts and talents, as our previous stories have illustrated. Like Sarah, you can utilize your passion and talents, coupled with the compassion cultivated through yoga, to contribute to societal change. Your yoga practice is not just a path to personal growth but a springboard for social activism and community engagement.

In the spirit of yoga, let's harness the power of compassion and act for social change. Remember, every small step counts. With yoga as our guiding philosophy, we can make a difference.

The Power of Compassion in Yoga

In this transformative journey, we've explored how compassion, a core principle of yoga, serves not only as a personal tool for growth but also as a catalyst for social change and activism. The stories we've shared highlight how compassion can emerge from the mat and into our communities, inspiring actions that resonate with our shared humanity.

Reflection: Your Compassionate Journey

As we conclude this chapter, reflect on your yoga journey so far. Has your practice evolved to include compassion, for yourself and others? How has it touched your life and possibly the lives of those around you? These reflections are important, not just as a measure of growth, but also as a stepping-stone to further cultivation of compassion.

Your Compassion Action Plan

To help you incorporate compassion into your daily yoga practice, here's an action plan template. Fill it out and refer back to it to remind yourself of your commitment:

1. **Compassion towards self:** Identify areas where you can be more compassionate towards yourself. Write down specific practices or actions to cultivate self-compassion.
2. **Compassion towards others:** List ways you can extend compassion to others in your daily life.
3. **Compassion for social change:** Identify one social issue that resonates with you. Outline actions you can take, using your yoga practice as a foundation, to contribute to this cause.

Remember, the goal is not to perfect these actions but to commit to a journey of continued growth, compassion, and change.

As we close this chapter, remember that compassion is like a muscle. It requires consistent practice to strengthen and grow. Yet, its power is transformative – for you, for those around you, and ultimately, for our shared society.

I look forward to our continued exploration in Chapter 15: The Power of Ritual in Yoga. Here, we'll delve into how incorporating rituals into our practice can deepen our connection, create sacred space, and mark our personal transformations. Let's continue this journey, together.

15

The Power of Ritual in Yoga

Rituals in Yoga: A Pathway to Deeper Connection

The power of ritual is universally recognized and respected across diverse cultures and traditions. In yoga, rituals play a significant role in enhancing the spiritual dimension of the practice, transforming it from merely a series of postures to a holistic journey of self-discovery and mindfulness. Incorporating rituals in yoga can deepen our connection to the practice, create a sacred space for personal growth, and mark our transformative journey.

Understanding Rituals in Yoga

Rituals in yoga are not about rigid rules or ceremonies but rather intentional practices that add a deeper layer of meaning and reverence to your yoga journey. They can be as simple as lighting a candle before starting your yoga practice, setting an intention, or chanting a mantra. The ritual could also be the act of rolling out your yoga mat in a designated, tranquil space in your home.

The essence of rituals lies not in the specific act itself, but in the mindful intention behind it. They serve as reminders to slow down, to stay present, and to approach the practice with respect and purpose. When infused with personal meaning, rituals create a bridge between the physical and the spiritual, grounding us in the moment and enhancing the transformative power of yoga.

Your Current Understanding of Rituals

Before we delve further into the subject, let's gauge your current understanding and usage of rituals in your yoga practice. Answer the following questions:

1. Do you have any specific rituals you currently follow before, during, or after your yoga practice? If yes, what are they?
2. How do these rituals enhance your yoga practice?
3. What meaning or intention do you attach to these rituals?
4. Are there any new rituals you would like to introduce to your practice?

This self-assessment is not an evaluation but rather a reflective exercise. It's an opportunity to introspect on your personal relationship with rituals in yoga and to identify areas you may wish to explore or deepen further.

Benefits of Incorporating Rituals into Your Yoga Practice

Rituals in yoga extend beyond the physical practice, anchoring us in mindfulness and intentionality. Let's explore some of the profound benefits of incorporating rituals into your yoga practice:

- **Creating a Sacred Space:** Rituals can help establish your yoga space as sacred, whether it's a corner of your bedroom or a dedicated yoga room. This sacred space serves as a sanctuary for your practice, cultivating a serene and focused atmosphere.
- **Cultivating Mindfulness:** Rituals, by their very nature, invite us to slow down, be present, and engage fully with the task at hand. This promotes mindfulness, which enhances both our yoga practice and overall well-being.
- **Deepening Connection:** Rituals can deepen our connection with the practice, our bodies, and our inner selves. They can act as powerful tools for self-discovery and personal growth.
- **Amplifying Intentions:** Rituals can help clarify and amplify our intentions. By beginning our practice with a clear intention, we imbue our movements and breaths with purpose, creating a more meaningful experience.
- **Marking Transitions:** Rituals can also serve as markers of transitions, both within the yoga practice (such as moving from a period of activity to relaxation)

and in our personal lives (such as marking a significant life event or personal accomplishment).

In the next sections, we'll explore specific rituals that you can incorporate into your yoga practice and how to create your own personal rituals. We'll also look at how rituals can enhance not only your practice but also your everyday life. Stay tuned, and let's delve deeper into the transformative power of rituals in yoga.

The Importance of Ritual in Yoga Practice

Diving Deeper into the Significance of Rituals

Rituals in yoga are more than just habits or routines; they are purposeful actions that imbue our practice with a deeper meaning. Incorporating rituals in yoga can create a more grounded, mindful, and focused atmosphere. By starting with an intentional ritual, we tune into our mind-body connection, reminding ourselves that our practice is more than just a physical workout—it is an inward journey towards self-discovery and balance.

Every time we roll out our mat, set our intention, or close our practice with a heartfelt Namaste, we're engaging in a ritual. These actions help us cultivate a profound connection with our practice, bringing a sense of reverence and mindfulness that resonates beyond the yoga mat and into our daily lives.

Personal Story: David's Transformation Through Ritual

Recall David's story. A successful lawyer, David felt overwhelmed despite his achievements. Yoga and meditation became his refuge from the pressures of work, providing him with much-needed peace and clarity. David soon realized that a significant part of this transformative power came from his pre-practice ritual of setting up his yoga space with a lit candle and incense. This ritual marked his transition from the chaos of the world to the tranquility of his mat.

David found that this simple act allowed him to create a sacred space for his practice, enhancing his focus and deepening his connection to yoga. This ritual didn't just transform David's yoga practice; it also spilled over into his professional life. He began to implement small rituals in his work, such as mindful breaks, which improved his stress management. David's story beautifully illustrates how rituals, as simple as they may seem, can have profound effects on our yoga practice and overall well-being.

Reflect on Your Own Practice

As we delve deeper into the importance of rituals in yoga, take a moment to reflect on your own practice. Here are some questions to guide your reflection:

1. Do you currently incorporate any rituals into your yoga practice?
2. How do these rituals impact your yoga experience?
3. Can you identify any new rituals you would like to introduce into your practice?

By recognizing the significance of rituals and mindfully incorporating them into your yoga practice, you can deepen your connection to your practice, further enhancing its transformative power.

Establishing a Personal Yoga Ritual

The Beauty of Personal Yoga Rituals

Yoga rituals aren't one-size-fits-all. They are deeply personal, reflecting our beliefs, intentions, and unique yoga journey. A personal yoga ritual is like a compass, guiding us into our practice with a sense of purpose and connection. From lighting a candle to reciting a mantra or even the sequence of asanas we choose—each element of our ritual becomes a sacred thread that weaves our practice into a beautiful tapestry of mindfulness, intention, and inner harmony.

Crafting Your Personal Yoga Ritual

Creating your own yoga ritual doesn't have to be complicated—it's about simplicity and authenticity. Your ritual should resonate with you, not merely mimic what others are doing. Here are some steps to help you create your personal yoga ritual:

1. **Set Your Intention:** Before you begin your practice, take a moment to reflect on your intentions. Do you wish to cultivate inner peace, enhance your focus, or perhaps open your heart to more compassion?
2. **Create Your Sacred Space:** Your environment matters. Choose a space where you feel comfortable and at peace. You can personalize this space with items that evoke tranquility and positivity for you—this could be a candle, crystals, incense, or even a favorite piece of artwork.

3. **Choose Your Ritual Elements:** Decide on elements that reflect your intention. These can be yoga postures, breathing exercises, meditation, or mantras. Remember, this should be something that resonates with you and helps anchor your intention.

4. **Seal Your Practice**: End your practice with a concluding ritual. This could be a moment of gratitude, a meditation, or even a simple "Namaste" to yourself. This helps seal in the benefits of your practice and signifies a respectful closure.

5. **Consistency:** While the elements of your ritual can change as you grow in your yoga journey, maintaining a consistent routine can deepen your connection to your practice. Remember, it's not about perfection but progression.

Design Your Personal Yoga Ritual Worksheet

To assist you in creating your personal yoga ritual, here's a worksheet layout you can use:

- **My Intention:** Write down what you wish to cultivate through your yoga practice.
- **My Sacred Space:** Describe your chosen space for yoga practice and how you wish to personalize it.
- **Ritual Elements:** List the elements you wish to include in your yoga ritual that reflect your intention.
- **Sealing My Practice:** Decide on how you would like to conclude your yoga practice.

Take your time with this worksheet, and remember, your personal yoga ritual should be a reflection of you—your beliefs, your intentions, and your journey. As you grow in your practice, you'll find that your ritual evolves with you, always serving as a beacon guiding you back to your mat and your authentic self.

Using Rituals to Deepen Your Yoga Practice

The Power of Ritual in Yoga

Yoga is more than a physical practice. It's a journey of self-discovery, a bridge connecting body, mind, and spirit. Rituals are an integral part of this journey. They not only anchor our practice but also infuse it with meaning, mindfulness, and intention. The beauty of rituals lies in their transformative power—they can transform a simple yoga session into a sacred experience, deepening our connection to the practice and ourselves.

Enhancing Your Yoga Practice with Rituals

Just like each yoga pose has its unique energy and purpose, every ritual you incorporate into your practice brings its own vibrancy. A ritual could be as simple as lighting a candle before starting your practice, or as profound as chanting a specific mantra during meditation. What matters is the intention behind it. Rituals remind us to be present, to focus, and to set our intentions, ultimately enhancing the depth and meaningfulness of our practice.

Practical Tip: Integrating Rituals into Your Practice

- **Start with Simplicity:** Begin with a simple ritual that resonates with you. It could be lighting incense, chanting a mantra, or even drinking a cup of herbal tea before your practice.

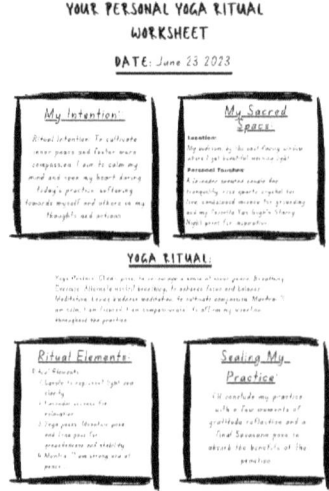

- **Set Your Intention:** Setting an intention is a powerful ritual that gives purpose to your practice. Take a moment before you begin to reflect on what you wish to cultivate or let go of during your practice.
- **Introduce Ritualistic Breathing:** Pranayama, or breath control, is a ritual itself. Techniques like Nadi Shodhana (alternate nostril breathing) or Kapalabhati (skull-shining breath) can help clear your mind and prepare your body for your practice.
- **Ritualize Your Asana Practice:** Whether you choose a vigorous Vinyasa flow or a peaceful Hatha sequence, be mindful of each movement, treating it as a sacred ritual.
- **End with Gratitude:** Conclude your practice by taking a moment to express gratitude—for your body, your breath, your practice, or anything else you feel grateful for. This ritual of gratitude can create a positive energy that extends beyond your practice.

Reflecting on Rituals

Here are some reflection questions to consider as you explore integrating rituals into your yoga practice:

1. What rituals are you already using in your yoga practice, even unknowingly?
2. What is your intention for integrating more rituals into your practice?
3. What rituals resonate with you and why?
4. How do you feel these rituals could deepen your connection to your practice?

Rituals in yoga aren't about routine—they're about reverence. They remind us that every breath we take, every pose we strike, every intention we set, is part of a larger, beautiful journey. By integrating rituals into our practice, we make each yoga session a mindful, intentional act, deepening not just our connection to the practice, but to our authentic selves.

Rituals for Special Occasions and Life Transitions

Celebrating Life's Milestones with Yoga Rituals

Yoga rituals hold a unique power to commemorate special occasions and assist us in navigating life transitions. They imbue these significant moments with mindfulness, reflection, and connection, helping us to fully experience, appreciate, and understand the change. For instance, a special yoga sequence on your birthday can symbolize growth and transformation, while a dedicated ritual when moving homes could represent letting go and embracing new beginnings.

Yoga Rituals for Special Occasions

Imagine waking up on your birthday and instead of rushing to start the day, you take time for a personal yoga ritual. This could involve a yoga sequence focused on gratitude and celebration, followed by a few moments of reflection on the year past and the year ahead. Such a ritual not only commemorates the day but also sets a positive and mindful tone for the coming year.

Navigating Life Transitions with Yoga

Transitions like moving homes, starting a new job, or experiencing the end of a relationship can be stressful. Yoga rituals can provide a comforting sense of stability and perspective during these times. You might create a ritual around grounding poses, like mountain or tree pose, to remind you of your strength and resilience amidst change.

Practical Tip: Crafting Your Special Occasion Ritual

- **Identify the Occasion or Transition:** What is the significant event you're marking? Understanding the nature of the occasion can guide your ritual creation.
- **Set an Intention:** Reflect on what this event signifies for you. What do you wish to cultivate or release?
- **Design Your Yoga Sequence:** Choose asanas that resonate with your intention. For instance, heart-opening poses for celebrations, or grounding poses for transitions.

- **Incorporate Meditation or Pranayama:** Consider including a specific breathwork technique or a themed meditation to deepen the impact of the ritual.
- **Finalize with a Closing Ritual:** Conclude your practice with a personal ritual—this could be expressing gratitude, journaling, or simply savoring a few moments of stillness.

Your Personal Yoga Ritual Planner

Consider the following elements when designing your personal yoga ritual:

- **Occasion or Transition:** (Describe the event or transition.)
- **Intention:** (What is your intention for this ritual?)
- **Yoga Sequence:** (List the asanas and their order.)
- **Breathwork/Meditation:** (Describe the breathwork technique or meditation theme.)
- **Closing Ritual:** (What will you do to conclude the ritual?)

This planner should be laid out in a linear sequence, with space provided after each prompt for readers to fill in their responses. You might include inspiring images or quotes alongside each section to further inspire and guide the reader.

By integrating yoga rituals into special occasions and transitions, we invite a deeper level of awareness and appreciation into our lives. These practices not only enhance our yoga journey but enrich our life journey, offering a sacred space for celebration, reflection, and growth.

Creating Sacred Space for Yoga and Meditation

The Sanctity of Space in Yoga and Meditation

Creating a dedicated space for yoga and meditation practices becomes a ritual in itself—one that reinforces your commitment and deepens your engagement with these practices. By crafting a space that is clean, calm, and personal, you create an environment that is conducive to inner exploration and peace.

Your sacred space doesn't have to be a separate room or a fancy corner with expensive equipment. It's a place where you feel safe, comfortable, and inspired, somewhere you can leave the busyness of the world behind and connect with your inner self.

Crafting Your Sacred Space: A Guide

A sacred space for yoga and meditation can be anywhere you choose, but there are a few considerations that can make the area more inviting and conducive to your practice. Here are some guidelines to help you craft your personal sanctuary:

- **Cleanliness and Orderliness:** Keep your space clean and free from clutter. A clean space encourages a clear mind, which is essential for effective yoga and meditation.
- **Lighting and Ambience:** Natural light is ideal, but if not possible, use soft and warm lighting to create a serene environment. Consider using candles or fairy lights to add a touch of warmth and charm.
- **Personal Items:** Personalize your space with items that inspire tranquility and positivity. It could be a favorite throw rug, a cherished photograph, or a meaningful keepsake.
- **Nature Elements:** Incorporating elements of nature can enhance the sense of tranquility in your space. This could include houseplants, a small water fountain, or natural stones.
- **Quietness:** Ideally, your space should be as quiet as possible. However, if that's not feasible, consider using noise-cancelling headphones or soft, ambient sounds to help maintain your focus.

Designing Your Sacred Space Template

Envisioning your sacred space is the first step to creating it. This template should be laid out as a list with ample space for readers to write their responses.

1. **Location:** (Where will your sacred space be located?)
2. **Cleanliness and Orderliness:** (How will you maintain cleanliness and order?)
3. **Lighting and Ambience:** (What type of lighting will you use? What additional elements could create a soothing ambience?)

4. **Personal Items:** (What personal items could make your space more comfortable and inspiring?)
5. **Nature Elements:** (How might you incorporate elements of nature into your space?)
6. **Sound:** (How will you manage the noise level in your space?)

Creating a sacred space for yoga and meditation is a personal and deeply rewarding journey. It's a testament to your commitment and respect for your practice, a sanctuary where you can leave the distractions of the world behind and connect with your true self.

Interactive Exercise: Designing Your Own Yoga Ritual

Crafting Your Personal Yoga Ritual

Creating your unique yoga ritual can be a rewarding journey of personal discovery. This exercise encourages creativity, self-expression, and an exploration of what yoga truly means to you. Let's design a ritual that brings positivity, calmness, and a profound sense of self-awareness to your daily life.

Step by Step: Designing Your Yoga Ritual

1. **Find your purpose:** Your ritual should revolve around a purpose or intention. It could be as simple as starting your day with positivity, or as deep as fostering spiritual growth.
2. **Choose your yoga sequence:** Depending on your purpose, choose a yoga sequence that resonates with you. This could be a calming sequence for stress relief or a dynamic sequence for energy and focus.
3. **Select your ritual elements:** Incorporating additional elements into your ritual can enhance the overall experience. This could be lighting a candle, playing calming music, or burning incense to create an atmosphere of tranquility.
4. **Decide the duration:** How long will your ritual be? A 5-minute morning routine or an hour-long end-of-day ritual? The duration should work for you, not against you.
5. **Plan the sequence:** Sketch out the sequence of your ritual. For instance, you might start with a moment of silence, followed by your chosen yoga sequence, and ending with a moment of gratitude.

Your Personal Yoga Ritual Worksheet

This worksheet is a guide for you to plan and document your personal yoga ritual. It's structured as a table with space for readers to fill in their responses, broken down into the following sections:

1. **Purpose:** (What is the intention behind your yoga ritual?)
2. **Yoga Sequence:** (What yoga poses will you include in your ritual? How will they be sequenced?)
3. **Ritual Elements:** (What additional elements will you incorporate into your ritual to enhance the experience?)
4. **Duration:** (How long will your ritual take? Will it change depending on the day or your mood?)
5. **Sequence of Ritual:** (In what order will you perform each element of your ritual?)

Remember, your yoga ritual is a personal expression of your journey with yoga. It should bring you joy, peace, and a sense of connection with yourself. Let your creativity flow, and enjoy the process of designing your own unique yoga ritual!

Yoga and Aromatherapy: Incorporating Essential Oils into Your Practice

The Scented Studio: The Power of Aromatherapy in Yoga

Incorporating aromatherapy into yoga is like adding a new dimension to your practice. The scents of essential oils can create an inviting atmosphere, evoke emotions, and even enhance your physical and mental performance. Yoga and aromatherapy are a powerful combination that can heighten your mindfulness, deepen your relaxation, and improve your overall well-being.

David's Story: An Aromatic Twist to Yoga

Remember David? The successful lawyer turned yoga enthusiast who used rituals to enhance his yoga practice and work-life balance? Well, David has another layer to his yoga journey that beautifully weaves in the power of aromatherapy.

In his quest to deepen his yoga practice and create a more serene environment, David decided to incorporate essential oils into his ritual. One day, he added a few drops of lavender oil to his diffuser during his evening yoga practice. The sweet, floral aroma filled his sacred space, and he instantly noticed a profound sense of calm sweep over him. His mind quietened, and he felt more present in his practice than ever before. This was a game-changer for David. Aromatherapy had heightened his yoga experience, and he made it a regular part of his practice.

Practical Tips: Choosing Essential Oils for Yoga

As you consider incorporating aromatherapy into your own yoga practice, it's essential to choose oils that resonate with your needs. Here are a few examples:

- **Lavender:** Known for its calming properties, lavender can help reduce stress and improve sleep. It's perfect for winding down in a relaxing evening yoga session.
- **Peppermint:** This refreshing scent can uplift your mood and increase focus, making it ideal for a morning yoga practice or anytime you need a mental boost.
- **Eucalyptus:** Eucalyptus oil can help clear the mind and promote relaxation. It's great for cooling down after a challenging workout or to help with deep, meditative breathing.
- **Sandalwood:** This earthy aroma is grounding and helps promote emotional balance, ideal for meditation or yoga sequences that emphasize stability and calm.

Incorporating essential oils into your yoga practice isn't just about choosing a pleasant fragrance. It's about selecting scents that align with your emotional and physical needs, enhancing your connection to your yoga practice. Try using them in a diffuser, adding a few drops to a warm bath before or after your yoga session, or even dabbing a bit onto your yoga mat.

The intertwining of yoga and aromatherapy can add a new depth to your ritual and make your practice even more rewarding. It's yet another way to make your yoga practice a uniquely personal journey of discovery and growth. As David learned, the right scent can elevate your practice to new heights. So, why not give it a try and see where these aromatic roads lead you?

The Transformative Power of Ritual in Yoga

As we close this chapter, let's reflect on the transformative power of rituals in yoga. Just as the deliberate arch of a cat's back in Cat Pose or the grounding of feet in Mountain Pose can deepen our practice, so too can the rituals we introduce into our yoga journey. Whether it's the calming scent of lavender before a meditative session or the savoring of herbal tea post-practice, these small, deliberate acts mark significant shifts, both within our bodies and minds, and in the greater context of our lives.

They help anchor us in the present, enhancing our sense of self-awareness, and facilitating personal growth. Rituals are like signposts on our yoga journey, marking significant milestones, and showing us how far we've come.

Your Yoga Ritual Action Plan

As an interactive element, I invite you to craft an action plan to incorporate rituals into your yoga practice. This is your chance to experiment and create a ritual that resonates with your unique needs and aspirations. Here are some steps to guide you:

- **Identify Your Intention:** What do you hope to achieve through your ritual? It could be a greater sense of calm, a deeper connection to your practice, or even marking a personal transition.
- **Choose Your Ritual:** The ritual should align with your intention. It can be as simple as lighting a candle or as complex as a series of asanas.
- **Implement Your Ritual:** Decide when and where you'll perform your ritual. Consistency is key, so try to make it a regular part of your yoga practice.
- **Reflect:** Over time, reflect on how your ritual is influencing your practice. Is it deepening your connection to yoga? If not, feel free to revise your action plan.

Reflect, Act, Anticipate

This chapter has illuminated how the transformative power of rituals can elevate our yoga practice. They are beautiful bridges between our yoga mat and our day-to-day life. As you start creating your Yoga Ritual Action Plan, I invite you to ponder these questions:

1. What part of my yoga practice feels most sacred to me?
2. How does the integration of rituals into my practice enhance my overall yoga experience?
3. What rituals might help me bring more of that sacredness into my everyday life?

And now, the invitation for action: implement your Yoga Ritual Action Plan in your next yoga session. Feel the shift as you engage more deeply, more mindfully.

Looking forward, we're about to embark on an exciting journey in Chapter 16: Yoga and Creativity: Unleashing Your Creative Potential. As we explore the profound connection between yoga and creativity, you'll learn to unlock the power of your creative spirit through your practice, transforming not just your yoga experience, but every aspect of your life.

Until then, may your practice continue to grow, and may your rituals bring you peace, clarity, and a deepened connection to your own personal yoga journey. Namaste.

16

Yoga and Creativity: Unleashing Your Creative Potential

Bridging Creativity and Yoga

As our exploration into the transformative power of yoga continues, we turn to an exhilarating intersection – yoga and creativity. Much like the rituals we've recently delved into, creativity is yet another intriguing facet of yoga, often overlooked but brimming with potential. Through yoga, we tap into an ancient wellspring of energy that can stimulate our creative thinking, driving us toward inventive expression and enriched life experiences.

Yoga doesn't merely enhance our physical strength and emotional balance; it also opens channels to our innate creative force. The link between yoga and creativity lies in their shared essence: a purposeful and wholehearted union of mind, body, and spirit. Both demand our presence, our dedication, and the courage to explore uncharted territories within us.

The Yoga-Creativity Connection: A Self-Assessment

To better understand your current relationship with creativity in yoga, let's pause for a moment and engage in a self-assessment.

1. How often do you feel a spark of creativity during or after your yoga practice?

2. Does your yoga practice inspire you to explore new ideas or projects outside of the mat?
3. Can you recall a time when an asana sequence triggered an imaginative thought or solution?

Take a few moments to consider these questions. There are no right or wrong answers – just insights into your unique interplay between yoga and creativity.

As we move forward, we'll delve deeper into how yoga can fuel your creative spirit, transforming not only your practice but also the way you perceive and interact with the world. As you ride the waves of your breath, you'll learn to navigate the seas of your creativity, uncovering treasures buried deep within your being. Are you ready to awaken the creative force within you?

Stay tuned as we venture further into this fascinating territory, where the realms of yoga and creativity converge. It's a journey that promises to be illuminating, inspiring, and deeply empowering. Namaste.

The Connection Between Yoga and Creativity

Yoga as a Catalyst for Creativity

Unbeknownst to many, yoga isn't merely a physical practice for fitness and flexibility. Instead, it is a holistic approach to overall wellbeing, stimulating our bodies, minds, and, surprisingly, our creative instincts.

Yoga is a potent tool to ignite the fires of creativity. Physically, the series of postures and movements improves blood flow, ensuring every cell, including those in our brain, are well-nourished. The consequent enhanced brain function paves the way for more novel, innovative thoughts.

Mentally and emotionally, yoga instills calm, making room for creativity to bloom. As the swirling storm of everyday worries dissipates, a tranquility settles, creating a fertile ground where creative seeds can sprout. The clarity fostered by yoga helps in recognizing and exploring these creative inclinations.

The Story of Paul: A Software Engineer turned Storyteller

Take Paul, an introverted software engineer, for instance. He spent his days buried in codes, convinced that creativity was for the 'artsy' types. That was until he discovered yoga.

Paul started practicing yoga to relieve his persistent backache. However, in the quiet moments of his yoga sessions, an unexpected guest appeared – stories. Images, characters, and plots started dancing in his mind. He began jotting these down, initially just to clear his head. However, he soon realized that his 'doodles' resonated with his friends' children. That's how Paul, the introverted software engineer, stumbled upon his latent talent for storytelling and embarked on a journey to become a children's book writer.

Reflect and Unleash Your Creativity

Consider your yoga practice. Has there been a moment, perhaps in the tranquility following a yoga session, when a creative idea flashed in your mind? Can you identify any change in your creative pursuits since you started practicing yoga? Reflecting on these questions might unveil surprising revelations about your creativity.

In summary, yoga nourishes creativity, letting it flow more freely. As Paul's journey shows, when you embrace yoga, you don't just gain physical strength and mental clarity. You might even discover a side of you that was hidden, waiting patiently to emerge and transform your life. Yoga can indeed be a key, opening the doors to your creative potential.

Yoga Poses and Practices for Boosting Creativity

Creativity isn't just about producing art; it's a way of thinking, a process that involves making connections and finding new solutions. It is the catalyst for innovation, problem-solving, and holistic well-being. And guess what? Yoga, with its emphasis on uniting mind, body, and spirit, can play a significant role in stimulating your creative instincts.

Embrace the Flow: Vinyasa Sequence

Vinyasa, or "flow," yoga can be particularly helpful in this regard. The smooth transitions and synchronized breathing encourage a mindful, focused state that can help release creative blocks and open up new channels of thought.

While you're likely familiar with some Vinyasa sequences, let's explore a few unique asanas to boost creativity. Remember, if a pose doesn't feel comfortable, adjust it, or use a yoga prop.

Lotus Pose (Padmasana)

While this pose is often used for meditation, it's an effective tool for sparking creativity as well. The alignment of the spine and the balanced, steady posture facilitate clearer thinking and a greater openness to new ideas.

Practical Tip: From a seated position, gently place your right foot on your left thigh and vice versa. Maintain a straight back, rest your hands on your knees with your palms facing up, and breathe deeply.

Gate Pose (Parighasana)

The Gate Pose offers a stretch that spans from your toes to your fingertips, engaging your mind and body in harmony. This deep, lateral stretch promotes a flow of energy throughout the body, freeing your creative instincts.

Practical Tip: From a kneeling position, extend your right leg out to the side. Reach your right arm down to your right leg, extend your left arm overhead and lean your torso towards the right. Hold for a few breaths, then repeat on the other side.

Goddess Pose (Utkata Konasana)

The Goddess pose embodies strength, power, and resilience. As you engage in this powerful standing pose, visualize yourself being filled with the same qualities, which can translate into confidence in your creative abilities.

Practical Tip: Stand with your feet wider than hip-width apart, turn your toes outwards, bend your knees, and lower your hips. Raise your arms to shoulder height and bend your elbows to form right angles, with your palms facing forward.

Embrace the Wild: Wild Thing (Camatkarasana)

The Wild Thing is an invigorating backbend that opens your chest, heart, and mind, unleashing your creative energy.

Practical Tip: Start in Downward-Facing Dog, lift your right leg and bend the knee, bringing your foot towards the left side of your body as you flip your hips to open into a backbend. Extend your right arm forward as if reaching for something. Remember to repeat on the other side.

Creativity-Boosting Yoga Sequence

Try this sequence: Begin with Lotus Pose for centering, transition into the Gate Pose to open your sides, move into the Goddess Pose to build strength and confidence, and finally, unfold into the Wild Thing pose to release your creative energy.

When you're done, lie down in Savasana, allowing your body to relax fully and your mind to absorb and integrate this new energy. As you lay there, let your mind wander freely. Don't force any creative thoughts, just allow them to come naturally. With regular practice, you might just find your creativity flourishing in unexpected ways.

Techniques for Tapping into Your Creative Flow

The creative flow isn't something you can simply summon at will—it's like a wild river, sometimes tranquil, sometimes turbulent, but always moving. As an avid yoga practitioner and meditator, I've spent years exploring ways to harmonize with this unpredictable current.

Dive into the Current: Yoga, Meditation, and Mindfulness

Yoga, meditation, and mindfulness aren't just about achieving physical flexibility or a calm state of mind. They offer gateways into our inner selves where the creative flow originates. Engaging in these practices can help you bypass mental barriers and tap into the river of creativity that flows within.

Yoga for Creative Flow

Yoga's ability to unite body, mind, and spirit offers a unique avenue into the creative process. As you move through asanas, focus on the rhythm of your breath, the sensation of your body moving, and let your mind enter a state of active meditation. This mindfulness can break down mental blocks and allow creative ideas to surface.

Mindfulness and Meditation

Mindfulness, the practice of being present and engaged in the moment, can help you tap into creativity by silencing the constant chatter of your mind, creating a fertile ground for fresh thoughts to grow.

Practical Tip: Start by selecting a quiet, comfortable place. Close your eyes and focus on your breathing, noticing the rise and fall of your chest. As thoughts come, acknowledge them without judgement, then let them go, returning your focus to your breath. With time and practice, this will create a space for creativity to thrive.

A Creative Flow Exercise

Let's get hands-on with an exercise designed to kickstart your creative flow. You'll need a pen and paper, a quiet space, and about 20 minutes.

1. Start with a few minutes of mindfulness meditation to clear your mind.
2. Now, think of a problem you've been struggling with, something that requires a creative solution.
3. Pose this problem to yourself, close your eyes, and perform a gentle yoga pose, like the Lotus Pose (Padmasana). As you hold the pose, focus on your breathing and the problem at hand.
4. Release the pose, sit comfortably, and start a 'free-writing' session for 10 minutes. Write anything and everything that comes to your mind about the problem, without worrying about grammar, punctuation, or making sense.
5. Once you're done, read through your writing. You might find seemingly unconnected ideas which, when viewed from a different perspective, can offer creative solutions.

Remember, accessing your creative flow isn't a one-and-done thing—it's a continuous journey. The more you practice these techniques, the more you'll find your creativity unblocked and flowing freely. Embrace this journey, trust in your unique creative process, and let the river of creativity guide you toward unexplored territories.

A Symphony of the Senses: Incorporating Art, Writing, and Music into Your Yoga Practice

Yoga has always been about unity, about bringing together body, mind, and spirit. It has a transformative potential that goes beyond the physical practice. By incorporating art, writing, and music into our yoga routines, we can tap into a deeper level of consciousness, creativity, and self-expression.

- **Yoga and Art:** A Canvas of Movement
- Art is a powerful medium of expression, of capturing the intangible and making it tangible. Much like yoga, it's a language that speaks from the soul.
- Think of your yoga mat as your canvas, and your movements as strokes of a brush. As you flow from one pose to another, imagine each motion leaving a trail of color behind. Visualizing this fusion of art and yoga can make your practice more dynamic and creatively stimulating.
- *Practical Tip:* Try sketching or painting after your yoga session. Use colors and forms to represent the energy, feelings, or thoughts that emerged during your practice. Don't worry about creating a masterpiece; the goal is to express, not to impress.
- **Yoga and Writing:** Inking Your Inner Dialogue
- Writing is a profound tool for reflection and self-discovery. It's a conversation with your inner self, just like yoga.
- Yoga can stir up a whirlpool of emotions, ideas, and thoughts. Writing after a session can help you channel these raw energies onto paper, gaining clarity and insights about your inner self.
- *Practical Tip:* Keep a yoga journal. After each session, write about your experience, emotions, thoughts, or any creative ideas that came to mind. This practice not only deepens self-awareness but also enhances your creativity.
- **Yoga and Music:** Harmonizing the Body and Mind

- Music, with its rhythm and melody, can enhance your yoga flow, synchronizing your movements and breath. It can also help transport you to a mental state conducive to creativity and imagination.
- *Practical Tip:* Create a yoga playlist that reflects the energy you want for your practice. This could be calm, instrumental tracks for a gentle session, or something more upbeat for a vigorous flow. Remember, the music should support your practice, not distract from it.

Reflection Questions

To further explore how art, writing, and music can be interwoven into your yoga practice, consider the following questions:

1. What emotions or images come to mind during your yoga practice? How could you express these through art?
2. How might writing after yoga sessions help you better understand your thoughts, feelings, or creative sparks that emerge during practice?
3. What type of music resonates with your yoga practice? How does it influence the energy, rhythm, or focus of your practice?

Yoga isn't confined to a sequence of poses—it's a living, breathing, creative practice that can encompass multiple forms of self-expression. By integrating art, writing, and music into your yoga, you can embark on a journey that transcends the physical, delving into a realm of enhanced creativity, deeper self-understanding, and boundless self-expression.

Guided Meditation: Awakening Your Creative Spirit

Unleashing your creative spirit starts from within. Our minds, often cluttered with thoughts, can benefit from the tranquility of meditation, making space for the spark of creativity to ignite. Let's embark on a journey to awaken your creative spirit through a unique guided meditation.

Creating a Conducive Environment

Practical Tip: Prior to starting your meditation, ensure you are in a peaceful environment. It should be free from distractions and noises. Comfort is key, so find a cozy spot, perhaps surrounded by objects that inspire you—art, nature, or anything that kindles your imagination. A little soothing background music can also aid relaxation. Remember, this is your sacred space to unleash your creativity.

Guided Meditation

Let's begin. Sit comfortably, close your eyes, and start by taking deep, calming breaths. As you inhale, visualize drawing in pure, creative energy. As you exhale, let go of doubt, fear, or any creative blocks.

The Journey Within: Envision a soft, warm light at your core. This light represents your creative spirit. See it radiate from within you, growing brighter with each breath.

The Flowing River: Now, imagine this light transforming into a gentle, flowing river. This river symbolizes your stream of creativity. Notice its depth, its pace. Is it a slow meandering stream or a vigorous rush of water? There's no right or wrong; it's uniquely yours.

The Creative Garden: Picture your river leading to a beautiful garden, the garden of your mind. It's fertile with ideas waiting to bloom. Walk in this garden, feel the possibilities, the growth, the creative potential.

Harvesting Ideas: Reach out and pluck an idea, visualized as a glowing orb. This is your creative offering, born from the depths of your creative spirit.

Cultivating Gratitude: Finally, hold this idea close to your heart and express gratitude. Gratitude for your unique creativity, for the ideas that you will bring into the world.

Return from your meditation journey by taking a few more deep breaths, bringing your awareness back to your surroundings. Open your eyes, carry this creative energy with you, and allow it to infuse into your daily life and actions.

By journeying within ourselves, we can tap into our creative reservoir, fostering a mindset that celebrates creativity and invites inspiration in all forms. This meditation can be a powerful tool to awaken and harness your creative spirit.

Interactive Exercise: Expressing Your Inner Light through Creative Exploration

Art, in its countless forms, is a beautiful medium to express your inner light. We all carry a unique, vibrant light within us - our passions, our strengths, our dreams. This exercise invites you to explore and express that light through creative exploration.

Creative Exploration Exercise

Practical Tip: You'll need your preferred art materials, an open mind, and a heart ready for self-expression. This can include paints, pens, clay, music instruments, or anything else that stirs your creative spirit.

- **Step 1: Finding Your Inner Light** - Start by closing your eyes and taking a few deep breaths. Visualize your inner light, an energy that is distinctly you. It could be a color, a shape, a sound, or a sensation.
- **Step 2: Expressing Your Light** - Open your eyes and start creating, letting your inner light guide your process. Don't worry about creating something "perfect." This is your safe space to express freely.
- **Step 3: Reflection** - After you've finished creating, take a step back. Observe what you've created and reflect on the experience. How does it feel to express your inner light? What have you learned about yourself in this process?

The Inner Light Worksheet

Design a simple worksheet with three sections titled "Visualization," "Expression," and "Reflection."

- **Visualization:** Note down what your inner light looks like. Is it radiant like a star, or gentle like a candle's glow? Maybe it's not a visual image at all, but a feeling or sound. There's no wrong answer.
- **Expression:** Here, describe your creative process. What medium did you choose, and why? What choices did you make as you were creating?
- **Reflection:** Write about your experience after the creative process. What did you discover about your inner light? How does it feel to see it represented through your art?

Use this worksheet every time you perform this exercise. It will document your journey, showing you how your inner light evolves over time, and how you grow along with it.

Remember, the goal is not to produce an artistic masterpiece, but to tap into your inner world, exploring and expressing the light within you. Embrace the process with an open mind and enjoy the beautiful journey of self-discovery.

Case Studies: Artists and Creatives Inspired by Yoga

Yoga and creativity often go hand-in-hand, with the mindfulness, self-awareness, and mental clarity cultivated through yoga frequently sparking artistic and creative breakthroughs. Let's look at a few case studies that exemplify this potent combination.

Emily's Artistic Revolution

Meet Emily, a graphic designer bogged down by the constraints of corporate design. She turned to yoga for stress relief, but found an entirely new approach to her art. Asana practice became a conduit for imaginative thoughts, flowing through her mind like a stream of colors. Yoga's emphasis on mind-body connection fostered Emily's artistic breakthrough, unleashing a style that was expressive, bold, and truly her own.

Joseph's Symphony of Serenity

Joseph, a classically trained musician, experienced a creative block. His music felt stiff and impersonal, disconnected from his own emotions. Then, he discovered yoga. The harmonious balance of movement and breath in yoga, the symphony of serenity it evoked, began to seep into his compositions. Yoga connected Joseph to his inner self, enabling him to compose music that was a true reflection of his spirit.

Personal Experiences: Testimonials

In Emily's words, "Yoga opened the floodgates of my creativity. The asanas unlocked my body, the meditation quieted my mind, and somewhere between, my artistic voice found its echo."

Joseph recounts, "Yoga taught me the beauty of balance, of rhythm, of harmony. These elements found their way into my music, making it not just a composition but an emotional expression."

Reflect and Apply

Let's bring this home. Consider these reflection questions:

1. How does your yoga practice stimulate your creativity?
2. What specific elements of yoga resonate with your creative work?
3. How can you further cultivate creativity through your yoga journey?

Remember, like Emily and Joseph, yoga can be more than just a physical practice. It can be a channel for creativity, a platform for self-expression, and a bridge to connect you with your unique, artistic self.

The Power of Yoga in Unleashing Creativity

As we bring Chapter 16 to a close, let's take a moment to honor the profound power of yoga in fostering creativity. This ancient practice, far more than a physical discipline, serves as a conduit for unlocking our inherent creativity, enabling us to reach new heights of inspiration and innovation.

Yoga and Creativity: A Transformative Union

Throughout this chapter, we've delved into the remarkable stories of individuals who tapped into their creative potential through the practice of yoga. From painters to writers, entrepreneurs to musicians, yoga has been a catalyst for these artists and creatives, empowering them to transcend limits and express their true selves.

Remember, creativity isn't confined to artistic pursuits; it's about problem-solving, innovating, and seeing the world from unique perspectives. Whether you're an artist or an engineer, a teacher or a scientist, yoga can awaken your creative essence and illuminate your unique talents.

Your Yoga-Creativity Action Plan

Now it's time for you to create your own Yoga-Creativity Action Plan. Take a piece of paper and outline your personal goals for integrating yoga into your creative process. What yoga techniques would you like to try? How might you schedule yoga into your routine to maximize your creative output?

Reflect on how yoga can enhance your creative pursuits and vice versa. Is there a particular creative endeavor you've been longing to explore, or a project you've felt stuck on? How might you use yoga to fuel your creative energy and find fresh inspiration?

Reflect, Act, and Look Forward

Reflect on the profound wisdom shared in this chapter. How might you weave these insights into your yoga practice and creative endeavors? Challenge yourself to try a new yoga pose or practice mindful breathing during your next creative session. Pay attention to the subtle shifts in your creative energy.

As we move towards the end of this chapter, I invite you to anticipate the journey ahead. In Chapter 17, we'll be 'Exploring Yoga Styles and Traditions', taking a deep dive into the rich tapestry of practices that make up the world of yoga. Prepare to expand your knowledge and ignite your curiosity as we uncover the depth and breadth of yoga's diverse styles and traditions.

Remember, the journey of yoga is about continuous growth and exploration. Yoga isn't just a tool for enhancing creativity; it's a journey towards self-discovery and a path towards a vibrant, balanced, and fulfilling life. So, take a deep breath, step onto your mat, and prepare to unleash your creativity through the transformative power of yoga.

17

Exploring Yoga Styles and Traditions

Welcome to Chapter 17, the next stage in our journey through the world of yoga and creativity. As we step off the mat from Chapter 16, where we discovered yoga as a catalyst for creativity, we now enter a realm rich in diversity and steeped in tradition.

A World of Styles: Embracing Yoga's Diversity

Yoga, like creativity, thrives on diversity. As we've seen, yoga empowers us to unlock our creative essence. Now, we're about to journey into the labyrinth of yoga styles and traditions, each with its own unique approach and philosophy. From the gentle fluidity of Hatha to the intense heat of Bikram, from the spiritual depth of Kundalini to the rigorous alignment of Iyengar, yoga's multifaceted nature offers us an array of avenues for exploration.

Just as you found your unique creative voice through yoga, remember that there's a yoga style that aligns with your unique self. As we navigate these myriad traditions, may you find the one that resonates with your heart, fuels your creative energy, and supports your journey towards self-discovery.

Know Your Yoga: An Interactive Prelude

Before we delve into these styles and traditions, let's test your current understanding of yoga's diversity. This interactive quiz is designed to gauge your familiarity with different yoga styles. It's a fun, enlightening way to establish where your knowledge stands, and to pique your curiosity for what's to come. Don't worry about getting every answer right - the aim is to learn and discover!

Interactive Quiz: How Well Do You Know Your Yoga Styles?

1. Hatha Yoga is often called the yoga of balance. What does Hatha mean in Sanskrit?

    A) Fire and Water

    B) Sun and Moon

    C) Mind and Body

    D) Light and Dark

2. Which style of yoga is known for its use of props and focus on precise alignment?

    A) Iyengar Yoga

    B) Kundalini Yoga

    C) Ashtanga Yoga

    D) Bikram Yoga

3. Ashtanga Yoga is characterized by a series of poses done in a specific sequence. What does Ashtanga mean in Sanskrit?

    A) Eight Limbs

    B) Flowing River

    C) Sacred Movement

    D) Eternal Cycle

4. Vinyasa Yoga is often referred to as "Flow Yoga" due to its smooth, flowing movements. Which of the following best describes a characteristic of Vinyasa Yoga?

    A) It focuses primarily on maintaining each pose for long durations.

B) It involves a sequence of poses that are synchronized with the breath.

C) It strictly adheres to a fixed set of poses in a specific order for each session.

D) It is usually practiced in a room heated to approximately 105°F (40.5°C).

5. Which style of yoga combines physical postures, breathing exercises, meditation, and chanting?

A) Restorative Yoga

B) Vinyasa Flow

C) Kundalini Yoga

D) Yin Yoga

Please note: the correct answers are 1B, 2A, 3A, 4B, 5C.

This interactive quiz aims to provide a fun and engaging way for readers to test their knowledge about various yoga styles while also learning new information. Quizzes like this can be a great way to make the learning process more interactive and dynamic.

An Overview of Different Yoga Styles and Traditions

Understanding Yoga Styles: A Panoramic View

Now that we've gauged our understanding of various yoga styles, let's take a step back and witness the stunning panorama that is the world of yoga. Like different hues on an artist's palette, each style of yoga adds a unique color to our practice and creativity, expanding our mind's canvas.

Hatha Yoga: The Foundational Flow
Hatha, the "yoga of balance," is often seen as the mother of all yoga styles. Rooted in the principle of harmonizing the sun (Ha) and moon (Tha) energies within us, Hatha is an excellent starting point for

beginners. It eases you into the world of yoga with its gentle postures, encouraging mindfulness and tranquility.

Iyengar Yoga: Precision and Alignment
Next, we have Iyengar, named after its founder B.K.S. Iyengar. This style emphasizes precision, alignment, and the use of props. If you are meticulous in your creativity and appreciate detail, this style might resonate with you.

Ashtanga Yoga: The Eight-Fold Path
Ashtanga, translating to "eight limbs" in Sanskrit, offers a dynamic and physically demanding practice. It is characterized by a fixed sequence of poses synchronized with breath. This style is akin to a disciplined artist, committed to refining their technique through consistent practice.

Vinyasa Yoga: The Art of Flow
Vinyasa, often called 'Flow Yoga', connects breath and movement in a dance-like sequence. If your creativity thrives on rhythm and spontaneity, Vinyasa might just be your dance partner in the yoga studio.

Kundalini Yoga: The Spiritual Awakening
Finally, Kundalini yoga is a blend of physical postures, breathing exercises, meditation, and chanting, with the aim of awakening the spiritual energy within. For those seeking to integrate a spiritual dimension into their creativity, Kundalini can serve as a guide.

Understanding Yoga Styles: A Panoramic View

Let's continue our journey, turning our gaze now to Yin Yoga and Restorative Yoga. Each, in its own way, brings a unique depth and perspective to our practice.

Yin Yoga: A Deep, Slow Practice for Flexibility and Relaxation
Yin Yoga invites us to slow down and turn inward. This practice consists of holding passive poses for longer periods to target the deep connective tissues. For creatives, Yin can offer a tranquil space to let the dust settle and allow new ideas to surface.

Restorative Yoga: Healing and Rejuvenation through Supported Poses

Then there's Restorative Yoga, a gentle, healing practice that uses props to fully support the body in each pose. Like a nurturing creative retreat, Restorative Yoga allows us to release tension and replenish our energy.

A Tapestry of Traditions: Comparative Yoga Chart

To help you navigate these various styles, here's a comparison chart that outlines their unique aspects:

YOGA STYLE	KEY FOCUS	IDEAL FOR
Hatha	Balance & Tranquility	Beginners & those seeking a calm practice
Iyengar	Precision & Alignment	Detail-oriented individuals & those recovering from injuries
Ashtanga	Dynamic & Disciplined Practice	Fit individuals & those seeking a structured routine
Vinyasa	Rhythm & Flow	Those who love movement & creativity
Kundalini	Spiritual Awakening	Those seeking a holistic & spiritual practice
Yin	Deep Stretch & Mindfulness	Those seeking to release tension & cultivate patience

Take a moment to reflect on these styles. Which one sparks your curiosity? Which one resonates with your creative self? Remember, there's no 'right' choice, only the one that feels right for you. As we delve deeper into each style in the coming sections, I invite you to remain open, just as we do when we step onto the mat or engage in our creative endeavors. The world of yoga is vast and rich, offering an inspiring spectrum of practices to fuel your creativity and enrich your life.

Detailed Exploration of Each Yoga Style

Hatha Yoga: A Comprehensive Practice for Mind, Body, and Spirit

Exploring the Foundations of Hatha Yoga

Hatha Yoga is often where many start their yoga journey. Hatha, in Sanskrit, signifies the union of opposites - 'ha' (sun) and 'tha' (moon). This yoga style cultivates balance and harmony, integrating mind, body, and spirit. With its slow pace and focus on basic postures, it's ideal for beginners and those seeking a calm practice.

Tina's Transformation: Finding Balance in Hatha Yoga

Let's revisit Tina, our resilient single mother from Chapter 4. Tina first discovered yoga through Hatha. Amidst the demands of life, she found solace on her yoga mat. "Hatha yoga brought a sense of equilibrium in my chaotic life," she recalls. "Each asana was an invitation to reconnect with myself, my breath, my body."

Hatha Yoga and You: A Guided Reflection

Reflect on Tina's journey with Hatha Yoga. Do you crave balance and tranquility in your life, much like Tina did? How might Hatha's slow, deliberate movements complement your unique pace and rhythm? Would you appreciate its focus on foundational postures and breathwork? If these aspects resonate with you, Hatha Yoga might be your perfect partner on your yoga journey.

Vinyasa Yoga: The Art of Flow and Movement

A Journey through Vinyasa Yoga

Vinyasa Yoga, also known as "flow yoga," is a dynamic practice known for its fluidity and dance-like movements. This style connects each posture to the next using breath, creating a seamless stream of poses that almost resemble a choreographed routine. Born from the Ashtanga Yoga tradition, Vinyasa Yoga was popularized in the West in the late 20th century, offering practitioners a vigorous yet meditative form of yoga.

With its emphasis on movement, strength, and flexibility, Vinyasa Yoga can benefit a broad range of individuals. The fast-paced nature can provide a great cardiovascular workout, making it an excellent choice for those seeking physical activity. Meanwhile, the synchronization of breath and movement cultivates mindfulness, bringing mental and emotional benefits.

Personal Story: Emily's Artistic Revolution

Emily, a talented graphic designer, faced the monotonous demands of corporate design. It was when she discovered Vinyasa Yoga that her creativity truly blossomed. She was captivated by the fluidity of the movements and the rhythm of her breath. Each practice felt like a dance, sparking her imagination in unprecedented ways. The way she moved her body on the mat began to influence how she moved her hand across the canvas. The vivacity of Vinyasa Yoga inspired Emily to break free from the rigid confines of her work, giving rise to an expressive, vibrant, and unique style. Vinyasa Yoga was not just a practice for Emily, but a catalyst for her artistic revolution.

Is Vinyasa Yoga Your Style?

Now, it's time for reflection. Do you enjoy continuous movement and rhythm in your physical activities? Are you seeking a balance between physical exertion and mental tranquility? Are you drawn towards practices that let you express yourself and tap into your creative energy? If you answered yes to any of these questions, Vinyasa Yoga might just be your match. Remember, the essence of yoga lies in exploration and personal growth. So, why not give Vinyasa Yoga a try? Its dance-like flow could be the change of pace you're seeking.

Ashtanga Yoga: A Structured and Challenging Practice

An Introduction to Ashtanga Yoga

Born in the warm and bustling heart of Mysore, India, Ashtanga Yoga is a system of yoga popularized by K. Pattabhi Jois during the 20th century. Imagine standing in a warm, serene studio, your bare feet firmly rooted on the mat. You're moving through a series of intricate poses, each flowing seamlessly into the next, your breath perfectly synchronized with each movement. This is Ashtanga Yoga. Rooted in ancient tradition, Ashtanga, which translates to 'eight limbs,' offers a physically demanding, deeply purifying practice focused on self-study.

Featuring a series of sequences, each performed in the same order, Ashtanga Yoga can be intense and challenging, but equally rewarding. Its structured nature allows practitioners to cultivate discipline and strength, physically and mentally. The intense flow generates heat in the body, detoxifying muscles and organs. This approach can be particularly appealing to those who enjoy a rigorous, structured practice and wish to achieve a deep, holistic integration of mind, body, and spirit.

For beginners, you can start with the Sun Salutation A, a fundamental sequence in Ashtanga Yoga. It begins with Mountain Pose, moves through Forward Bend and Plank Pose, transitions into Four-Limbed Staff Pose and Upward Dog, and concludes with Downward Dog. These movements help build strength and flexibility while grounding you in the structured practice of Ashtanga.

Tina's Journey to Ashtanga

Remember Tina, the single mother we met earlier who found balance in Hatha yoga and practiced Kapalabhati for life's demands? She felt a need for something more rigorous, a practice that could challenge her and strengthen her resilience. That's when she found Ashtanga.

"For me, Ashtanga was like a dance - structured, rhythmic, and intensely beautiful," Tina shares. "It was physically demanding, yes, but with every sequence, I felt stronger, more disciplined. I started sleeping better, my digestion improved, and my energy levels soared. It was like a total body cleanse."

Is Ashtanga Your Path?

Do you enjoy routine and structure? Do you find strength in discipline? Are you seeking a holistic practice that challenges you physically and mentally, promoting detoxification and invigorating energy? If so, Ashtanga Yoga could be the right path for you. Reflect on what you're looking for in your yoga journey and consider trying a class. Remember, every practice starts with the first step.

Iyengar Yoga: Precision and Alignment for a Balanced Practice

Unveiling the Iyengar Yoga

Iyengar Yoga, named after its pioneer B.K.S. Iyengar, is a practice rooted in precision and alignment. Originated in the mid-20th century, it emphasizes on meticulous postural alignment, timing in poses, and the use of props for a balanced practice. The practice's structure allows students to delve into the intricacies of each pose, inviting a sense of mindfulness and inner harmony.

Who is it for?

Iyengar Yoga is suitable for anyone seeking a methodical, disciplined approach to yoga, focusing on alignment and form. It's an excellent choice for beginners due to its emphasis on proper posture, and can be highly beneficial for individuals recovering from injuries or managing chronic conditions.

Joseph's Encounter with Iyengar Yoga

Let's step into the shoes of Joseph, a classically trained musician who found himself in a creative rut. Disconnected from his emotions, his compositions felt rigid and impersonal. Then, he discovered Iyengar Yoga.

The practice, with its rhythmic discipline and attention to detail, resonated with Joseph. The precise nature of Iyengar mirrored his musical training, but the emphasis on personal awareness and internal balance was transformative. "It was like a symphony of serenity," he recollects. "I found myself in the music again, my compositions now mirroring my spirit."

Reflection Time: Is Iyengar Yoga Right For You?

Consider your current exercise routine. Are you more drawn to methodical, structured practices, or do spontaneous, fluid movements attract you? Do you appreciate the beauty of the minutiae, the intricacies of alignment, and precision? If your responses lean towards the former, Iyengar Yoga might just be the perfect path for you on your wellness journey.

Yin Yoga: A Deep, Slow Practice for Flexibility and Relaxation

Unraveling the Essence of Yin Yoga

Originating from Taoist philosophy, Yin Yoga, an antithesis to Yang, invites us to slow down and dive deep. Here, the emphasis is on cooling and relaxing the body. The poses, primarily targeting the connective tissues, are held for a longer duration - usually 3 to 5 minutes, or even longer. The beauty of Yin lies in its surrendering nature; it encourages you to let go and release the tensions.

Who Is Yin Yoga For?

Yin Yoga is especially beneficial for those leading fast-paced lives and seeking respite. If you're looking for improved flexibility, stress relief, and a deeper connection with your inner self, Yin could be your answer.

James's Yin Experience

Meet James, a marathon runner we met earlier. When he injured his knee, he was introduced to Yin Yoga as part of his rehabilitation. As he started holding poses longer, he found a deep sense of release, not only physically but also mentally. "It was like therapy," James reflects, "the focus on breathing and stillness taught me patience, resilience and helped me connect to a part of myself I never knew existed."

Reflection Time: Is Yin Yoga Your Path?

Reflect on your current routine - is it filled with movement and dynamism, leaving you craving some stillness? Do you wish to explore a quieter, introspective side of your practice? If you resonate with these, Yin Yoga could offer you the balance you seek. It's time to slow down and listen to what your body has to say.

Restorative Yoga: Healing and Rejuvenation through Supported Poses

Unveiling Restorative Yoga

Restorative Yoga is a gentle, healing practice designed to allow the body and mind to completely relax and restore. Developed in the mid-20th century by B.K.S. Iyengar, it involves passive stretching with the use of props for support, encouraging a deeper state of relaxation.

Is Restorative Yoga for You?

Do you crave relief from stress, anxiety, or aching muscles? If the answer is yes, the nurturing environment of Restorative Yoga could be your sanctuary.

Linda's Journey with Restorative Yoga

Let's turn to Linda, who we first met when she started using deep belly breathing to manage her anxiety and depression. After discovering the transformative effects of breathwork, she delved into Restorative Yoga. "In each pose, I felt my worries melting away," she says. "I was no longer a victim of my mental health but an active participant in my healing."

Reflection Time: Does Restorative Yoga Resonate with You?

Ask yourself: Does the idea of deeply relaxing, restorative postures appeal to you? Can you picture yourself sinking into a peaceful state of surrender, allowing your body to gently stretch and release? If this stirs a feeling of calm within you, then Restorative Yoga could be the soothing balm your soul yearns for. It's time to embrace tranquility and restore harmony.

Kundalini Yoga: Awakening the Energy Within

An Introduction to Kundalini Yoga

Kundalini Yoga, often called the "Yoga of Awareness," is an ancient practice that centers around awakening your inner energy. Originating from the Tantric tradition, it blends physical postures, breathwork, meditation, and mantra chanting, aiming to elevate your consciousness and promote self-awareness.

Who is Kundalini Yoga For?

Those seeking a holistic practice that encompasses physicality, spirituality, and mindfulness might find Kundalini Yoga a rewarding experience. It is ideal for anyone eager to explore their inner strength and the mysteries of the mind.

Alex's Transformation Through Kundalini Yoga

We've previously met Alex, an empathetic engineer who found fulfillment in helping others at a community center. When Alex started practicing Kundalini Yoga, his life took an unexpected turn. "It was like awakening a dormant part of myself," he shares. "The dynamic movements, deep breathwork, and the enchanting mantras ignited an inner strength I never knew I had. It empowered me to embrace my empathy and use it as a source of strength."

Reflection Point: Is Kundalini Yoga Your Path?

Reflect on this: Does the blend of physical and spiritual elements in Kundalini Yoga resonate with you? Are you intrigued by the idea of tapping into your dormant energy and finding an inner transformation? If you feel a spark of curiosity or interest, perhaps it's time to explore Kundalini Yoga – the gateway to your inner self.

Anusara Yoga: Celebrating the Heart and the Goodness Within

Delving into Anusara Yoga

Anusara yoga, founded by John Friend in 1997, embodies the essence of "flowing with grace." Its core philosophy cherishes life and the innate goodness within each of us. This yoga style goes beyond mere physical flexibility, focusing on emotional and spiritual development through its 'Universal Principles of Alignment.'

Anusara is an ideal choice for those who wish to blend a rigorous practice with a heart-centered philosophy. It inspires practitioners to explore their self-expression while emphasizing the alignment of poses, nurturing both physical posture and mental wellness.

Meet Benjamin: Transformation through Anusara

Our new companion on this journey is Benjamin, a hard-working journalist always chasing deadlines. Finding balance was a struggle until he chanced upon Anusara yoga. "It was as if I'd been thrown a lifeline," Benjamin reflects. "Anusara, with its unique blend of rigorous physical practice and gentle, heart-centric philosophy, was a revelation. Every session was like peeling layers, getting closer to my true self. It taught me that strength isn't just about the body; it's also about the mind and the spirit."

Is Anusara Your Style?

If you're intrigued by the concept of nurturing your heart while challenging your body, Anusara might just be the yoga style you've been looking for. Reflect on this: do you appreciate a structured approach to alignment? Does the blend of physical and emotional exploration resonate with you? If so, Anusara yoga may be the perfect addition to your wellness journey. Remember, every yoga journey is personal and unique. Embrace the exploration.

Power Yoga: A Strength-Building and Empowering Practice

Exploring Power Yoga

Power Yoga, a dynamic offshoot of Ashtanga Yoga, carries forward Ashtanga's high energy, synchrony of breath and movement, but it drops the rigid structure of sequence. Born in America in the 90s, Power Yoga, with its fitness-centric approach, offers an intense workout that promotes strength, flexibility, and stamina. It provides a physically challenging yet deeply empowering experience.

Personal Story: Unleashing Inner Power with Ethan

Meet Ethan, a diligent software developer who struggled with work-related stress. Intrigued by Power Yoga's physicality, he gave it a try. "Power Yoga not only sculpted my body, but it also built my mental strength," Ethan shares. "Each session pushed me to my limits, transforming each challenge into an accomplishment. It has become my personal fortress of resilience and strength."

Reflection Questions

Are you looking for a physically engaging practice that also bolsters your mental strength? Does a vigorous, fast-paced workout resonate with your fitness aspirations? If you identify with Ethan's journey, Power Yoga could be your next step towards self-empowerment. Reflect on these questions as you continue exploring your yoga journey.

Prenatal Yoga: Supporting Expectant Mothers on Their Journey

Born out of the need to support expecting mothers, Prenatal Yoga offers gentle, nurturing, and beneficial routines designed specifically for different stages of pregnancy. This style provides relief from discomfort, enhances body strength and flexibility, promotes relaxation and deep connection with the unborn child.

Personal Story: Mary's Journey

When Mary found herself pregnant with her first child, the physical and emotional changes overwhelmed her. Turning to Prenatal Yoga, she discovered a realm of calm and self-confidence. "Each pose brought me closer to my unborn baby," Mary reflects. "It helped me embrace the transformation of my body and prepare for the journey of motherhood. This practice has been my rock in these challenging times."

Reflection Questions

Are you or a loved one going through the transformative journey of pregnancy? Do you need a gentle and nurturing practice that supports your changing body and helps prepare for childbirth? If Mary's journey resonates, Prenatal Yoga might be your perfect companion. Reflect on these questions to explore if this practice aligns with your current stage of life.

Chair Yoga: Adapting Yoga for Different Abilities and Needs

The Essence of Chair Yoga

Born from the roots of classic Hatha Yoga, Chair Yoga was created to make the enriching world of yoga accessible to everyone, regardless of physical limitations or mobility issues. At its core, Chair Yoga encourages the same mindful movement, deep breathing, and mental focus as other yoga styles, but modified to use a chair for support, allowing practitioners to experience the benefits without strain.

Discovering Strength in Adaptation: Sam's Story

Let's meet Sam, a retired office worker with arthritis. His journey to yoga was unconventional and transformative. Discovering Chair Yoga was his turning point. The tranquility of the room, the sturdy comfort of the chair, and the gentle stretching of his body created an ambiance that was both serene and rejuvenating. "In the beginning, I was skeptical," he admits, "but Chair Yoga was different. It was gentle, soothing and most importantly, adaptable. With each session, I felt stronger, more flexible, and more confident. It gave me a new lease on life when I needed it the most."

Contemplating Chair Yoga: Is It Right for You?

Reflect on these questions: Do you feel a physical yoga practice is out of your reach due to age, illness, injury or disability? Are you seeking a gentle, adaptable yoga practice that still offers mental and physical benefits? If you answered yes to any of these, Chair Yoga might just be the accessible and transformative practice you're searching for. Remember, the essence of yoga is unity of mind, body, and spirit, and this essence remains unchanged, whether we practice on a mat or a chair.

Aerial Yoga: Taking Your Practice to New Heights

The Essence of Aerial Yoga

Aerial Yoga, or AntiGravity Yoga, is an exciting blend of yoga, dance, Pilates, and acrobatics, all performed with the aid of a hammock. Suspended above ground, practitioners explore traditional yoga poses with a new, liberating dimension. Introduced in the early 2000s by Christopher Harrison, this style encourages flexibility, balance, and strength. This playful yoga style may seem daunting initially, but it's suitable for anyone looking for an unconventional way to improve their fitness and challenge their boundaries.

The Skyward Journey of Rose

Enter Rose, a seasoned ballet dancer. Encountering the limitations of age and an injury, she felt her passion waning. Aerial Yoga, with the hammock's silk wrapped securely around her, holding her aloft in a serene dance of air and gravity, brought a sense of freedom that rekindled her spirit. However, Aerial Yoga rekindled her spirit. "The hammock was like a dance partner, supporting me, allowing me to explore movements I thought were no longer possible. I felt freedom, youthfulness, and exhilaration I hadn't felt in years."

Reflecting on Aerial Yoga

Consider these questions: Do you crave a creative twist to your physical routine? Does the idea of defying gravity excite you? If yes, Aerial Yoga might be the leap you need to elevate your yoga journey.

Making an Informed Decision: Choosing the Right Yoga Style for You

Assessing Your Needs and Goals

Finding the right yoga style is akin to finding the right pair of shoes – it should fit comfortably and cater to your unique needs and aspirations. Are you seeking physical vigor or mental tranquility? Is it injury recovery or spiritual exploration that draws you to yoga? The answers to these questions are the first stepping-stones towards identifying the yoga style that resonates with you.

Practical Tip: Factors to Consider

6. **Physical Health and Fitness:** If you're a seasoned athlete, styles like Power Yoga or Ashtanga might engage you. Both demand a high level of physical prowess and share a similar focus on flowing, dynamic movement as seen in Ashtanga's set sequence of postures. For those seeking gentle movements or dealing with injuries, Restorative or Chair Yoga could be suitable.
7. **Mental Well-being:** Looking for stress relief? Try Hatha or Yin Yoga. Seeking deeper self-awareness? Kundalini might be your path.
8. **Lifestyle:** Busy schedules might favor shorter, intensive sessions like Bikram Yoga, while those with more time might enjoy the slow pace of Iyengar.
9. **Personal Preference:** Enjoy working in a group? Try Vinyasa. Prefer solitary practice? Ashtanga's self-led style might be for you.

Your Yoga Selection Worksheet

Your Goal: [Physical Fitness/Stress Relief/Spiritual Growth]

Your Schedule: [Flexible/Busy]

Preference: [Group/Solo, Intense/Gentle]

Health Considerations: [Injuries, Age, Fitness Level]

Rate yoga styles you're interested in, based on these factors. A perfect match will feel like coming home, so listen to your intuition. The journey of yoga is personal. Remember, the goal isn't to perfect a pose but to unite your body, mind, and spirit in harmony.

Interactive Exercise: Exploring Different Yoga Styles

Dipping Your Toes In

Yoga is a smorgasbord of styles and experiences, and the best way to find your preferred flavor is to taste-test! Whether you try a Vinyasa class one day and Restorative the next, or switch from Ashtanga to Kundalini, this exercise is all about exploration. Experimenting with different styles is like stepping into an array of different worlds - each with its own charm and challenges.

For instance, in a Vinyasa class, try the Sun Salutation sequence for a dynamic flow of postures, or in a Yin Yoga class, explore the Butterfly pose to tap into the style's calming nature.

Practical Tip: Open Mind, Open Heart

Approach this exploration with curiosity and openness. Don't be discouraged if a style doesn't resonate initially. Often, it's the challenging or unfamiliar practices that offer the most room for growth. Remember, there's no 'one-size-fits-all' in yoga - only what serves you best in the present moment.

Reflection Journal

Returning to our journaling practice, document your yoga adventures. After each class, make a note of the style, your experiences, and feelings. Consider these prompts:

1. **Style and Instructor:** Which style did you try? Who guided your practice?
2. **Physical Response:** How did your body react during and after the session?
3. **Emotional and Mental States:** How did this style influence your emotions and thoughts?
4. **Affinity and Discomfort:** Which aspects were enjoyable or challenging?

By noting these reflections, you not only document your journey but also begin to discern the yoga style that truly aligns with your needs and goals. In yoga, as in life, the joy is in the journey, not the destination.

The Power of Diversity in Yoga

A Universe Within

As we close this chapter, it's clear that yoga isn't a one-way street, but a vibrant, ever-changing cosmos of possibilities. Exploring different styles is like journeying through this universe, each one offering a unique, enriching perspective. Every style serves as a powerful reminder of the strength in diversity and the beauty in unity that underpins the practice of yoga.

Mapping Your Yoga Voyage

To further your explorations, create an action plan. Jot down the styles you'd love to delve deeper into, the instructors that inspire you, and the classes or studios you want to visit. This action plan will act as your compass, guiding you through your diverse yoga voyage.

Reflect and Recalibrate

Pause here. Reflect on the experiences and insights gained in this chapter. How have these different styles impacted your yoga practice? What transformations have you noticed in your physical, emotional, or mental state?

Action Plan: The Journey Continues

Take your first step into the next phase of your yoga journey now. Sign up for that Ashtanga class you've been curious about, or try a home practice of Yin yoga. Whatever you choose, step on your mat with an open heart and a vibrant spirit.

Coming Up: Immersion Experiences

Our yoga journey is about to go deeper. In the next chapter, we'll explore workshops, retreats, and yoga teacher training. These experiences offer immersive journeys into yoga, providing opportunities for profound growth and transformation. As we close this chapter, remember the power of diversity in your yoga practice. It's the myriad of experiences and styles that makes our journey unique, enriching, and truly our own. As you step off the mat today, carry with you the understanding that yoga, in all its beautiful diversity, is a mirror of life itself, reflecting the strength in unity and the power in diversity. Here's to the journey ahead!

18

Yoga Workshops, Retreats, and Teacher Training

Welcome, my fellow yogi, to the next chapter in our voyage - Chapter 18. As we turn a new leaf, let's carry forth the lessons we've learned about the diverse and captivating world of yoga styles. Remember the unity in diversity we celebrated in our last chapter? Today, we're about to embark on a more immersive journey, one that takes us deeper into the realms of yoga.

Think of yoga as a garden, blossoming with diverse flowers, each representing a yoga style. Until now, we've explored these styles, acknowledging their unique beauty and scent. Now, imagine becoming a gardener of this landscape - getting your hands into the soil, nurturing the blossoms, and watching them flourish under your care. This is what our next phase is about - diving deeper, getting involved, and immersing ourselves fully into the nurturing essence of yoga.

In this chapter, we're going to explore yoga workshops, retreats, and teacher training. These immersive experiences are for anyone wishing to deepen their understanding and broaden their horizons. They're not limited to those wishing to teach yoga, but are also for those of us wanting to enrich our practice and learn more about this ancient discipline.

Let's begin with workshops. Yoga workshops are short, focused sessions that delve into specific aspects of yoga. Ever wanted to perfect your Warrior Pose or deepen your meditation technique? A workshop can guide you there. Workshops offer an opportunity to learn from experienced instructors, ask questions, and receive personalized feedback - invaluable assets on our yoga journey.

Yoga retreats, on the other hand, are like taking a plunge into a yoga-filled oasis. They offer an escape from the daily hustle and bustle, a chance to reconnect with ourselves in tranquil and often natural settings. Picture practicing Sun Salutations as the sun rises over a tranquil beach, or meditating in a lush forest, cocooned by the symphony of chirping birds and rustling leaves. These are not mere fantasies, but realities waiting to be explored in yoga retreats.

Lastly, we come to yoga teacher training - the pinnacle of immersion experiences. This is where you'll delve deep into yoga's philosophy, anatomy, and teaching methodology. Even if teaching isn't your ultimate goal, this training will transform your practice, deepen your understanding, and foster personal growth in unexpected ways.

With the courage of a pioneer and the heart of a yogi, let's dive into the depth of these experiences, each promising growth, transformation, and a deeper connection to your yoga practice. It's an exciting journey, and I'm thrilled to navigate these waters with you. So, let's get started, shall we?

1. What is a Yoga Workshop?

    A. An intense workout session

    B. A focused session exploring specific aspects of yoga

    C. A week-long retreat

2. What would you most likely experience in a Yoga Retreat?

    A. Guided tours of yoga studios

    B. Focused study on one yoga pose

    C. Immersive yoga practice in tranquil settings

3. Which of the following best describes Yoga Teacher Training?

    A. A quick course to learn yoga basics

    B. A deep dive into yoga philosophy, anatomy, and teaching methodology

    C. A daily yoga class

4. Who can benefit from attending Yoga Workshops, Retreats, and Teacher Training?

    A. Only those who want to become yoga teachers

    B. Only experienced yoga practitioners

    C. Anyone wishing to deepen their understanding and practice of yoga

5. What is one common benefit of attending Yoga Workshops, Retreats, or Teacher Training?

    A. They guarantee a job as a yoga instructor

    B. They promise to make you a yoga master instantly

    C. They provide immersive experiences that foster personal growth and deepen understanding of yoga

Remember, there are no "wrong" answers, but the quiz is intended to reflect your current understanding and perhaps highlight areas where you might want to focus more as we dive deeper into each of these experiences

Understanding the Benefits of Yoga Workshops and Retreats

Let's plunge into the sea of benefits that yoga workshops and retreats offer. As the waves of yoga knowledge, experience, and practice come rolling in, they shape us into better yogis and, indeed, better humans. Yoga workshops and retreats provide unique opportunities to deepen our understanding, refine our practice, and truly connect with our inner selves. They are an immersion into the world of yoga, where we can absorb every aspect of this holistic practice.

Deepening your Practice and Understanding through Workshops

Yoga workshops act as a magnifying glass, enabling us to focus on specific aspects of yoga that are of particular interest to us. For instance, if you've been curious about inversions but find them intimidating, a workshop dedicated to them can give you the necessary guidance and confidence. If you've ever wanted to delve into the philosophies that underpin yoga, a theory-based workshop can provide insight. These workshops often attract people with similar interests, creating a supportive community to learn and grow with.

Anecdote from a Yoga Practitioner: Ethan's Transformation

Recall Ethan, the software developer we met in an earlier chapter, who was struggling with work-related stress. After embracing Power Yoga, he discovered a workshop on yoga and stress relief. This workshop offered a deeper understanding of how yoga helps manage stress, highlighting specific poses and breathing exercises beneficial for stress relief. Attending the workshop, Ethan not only enriched his personal practice but also felt a profound shift in his perspective on stress management, providing him a toolkit to navigate his demanding work environment more resiliently.

Immersing in the Yoga Lifestyle through Retreats

Yoga retreats are like an extended yoga hug! They offer an immersive experience that allows us to disconnect from our everyday lives and reconnect with our inner selves. Retreats offer a harmonious blend of yoga practice, meditation, healthy food, and often beautiful natural environments. They present an opportunity to deepen our practice, nurture our bodies, and nourish our souls, while also connecting us with a community of like-minded individuals.

Reflection on the Mat: Is a Yoga Retreat for You?

1. Do you crave a deeper connection with your yoga practice?
2. Are you seeking a community of like-minded yogis to share your journey with?
3. Do you feel the need to disconnect from your daily routines and reconnect with your inner self?
4. Are you open to exploring yoga beyond the physical asanas, embracing meditation, yoga philosophy, and holistic living?
5. Would you enjoy yoga in the heart of nature, breathing in the freshness of a forest, or absorbing the tranquility of a beach?

These are not prerequisites but rather guiding questions to help you gauge if a yoga retreat could be the next step in your journey. Remember, the yoga path is personal, and it's all about what feels right for you.

In the end, both workshops and retreats offer unique avenues for growth. They help us navigate our yoga journey with a deeper understanding, fostering a bond with our practice that goes beyond the mat. As we delve into these experiences, we expand our yoga horizons and enrich our own lives and potentially the lives of those around us. So, with an open heart and an open mind, let's continue to explore these opportunities together.

How to Choose the Right Yoga Workshop or Retreat

Embarking on a yoga journey is a deeply personal endeavor, reflecting a commitment to personal growth, balance, and self-understanding. This journey's intensity and path differ from person to person, defined by individual needs, goals, and circumstances. Whether you decide to deepen your practice through a workshop or take a healing plunge with a retreat, making the right choice involves a few essential considerations.

Understanding Your Intentions

The first step in selecting the appropriate yoga workshop or retreat is understanding your intentions. Is there a specific aspect of your practice you wish to delve deeper into? Are you yearning for a transformational experience away from your daily routine, or do you seek focused learning on a particular yoga style or technique? The clarity of your intention can significantly influence your decision.

For instance, Emma, a high-powered executive, attended a weekend workshop on pranayama (breathwork). She sought to balance her fast-paced lifestyle, and this focused session offered her the tools to manage stress and reconnect with herself. On the other hand, Benjamin, the hard-working journalist, opted for a week-long Anusara yoga retreat. He needed a holistic experience to help him find equilibrium in body, mind, and spirit.

Assessing Your Availability

Another essential factor to consider is time. A yoga workshop can last for a few hours to a whole day, making it ideal for those with limited time. A yoga retreat, however, is an immersive experience that typically spans several days, requiring a more significant time commitment. Choose based on what suits your schedule without causing unnecessary stress or strain.

Evaluating Your Budget

Financial considerations also come into play. Workshops can be cost-effective, particularly if they are local. Retreats often come with a higher price tag due to accommodations, meals, and additional activities, but they offer a richer and more immersive experience. Remember, investing in your well-being is priceless, but it should also be balanced with your financial capabilities.

Understanding the Facilitators

Take a close look at who will be facilitating the workshop or retreat. Do their teaching style, philosophy, and values align with yours? A teacher's knowledge and approach can make a significant difference in your experience.

Researching facilitators can begin with reading their bios on workshop or retreat websites. Look for information about their yoga training, years of experience, and any specialties they may have. Do they have positive testimonials from previous participants? You can also see if they have published content online - articles, blogs, or videos - which can give you a sense of their teaching style and philosophy. Social media platforms can be helpful too, where they might share insights, thoughts, or class snippets.

Practical Tip: Research and Reflect

Take the time to research available options. Look at the course or retreat content, facilitators, location, duration, and cost. Reflect on your intentions, availability, and financial capacity.

Your Decision-Making Worksheet

To aid your decision-making process, here's a simple worksheet. Note down your findings and reflections as you research potential workshops or retreats:

1. Intention for attending a workshop or retreat:
2. Available time commitment:
3. Budget considerations:
4. Potential workshops or retreats:
5. Facilitator's teaching style and philosophy:

6. Final choice and reasoning:

YOGA WORKSHOP/RETREAT DECISION WORKSHEET

1. INTENTION FOR ATTENDING A WORKSHOP OR RETREAT:
   _____
   _____
   _____

2. AVAILABLE TIME COMMITMENT:
   _____
   _____
   _____

3. BUDGET CONSIDERATIONS:
   _____
   _____
   _____

4. POTENTIAL WORKSHOPS OR RETREATS:
   _____
   _____
   _____

5. FACILITATOR'S TEACHING STYLE AND PHILOSOPHY:
   _____
   _____
   _____

6. FINAL CHOICE AND REASONING:
   _____
   _____
   _____

Remember, every journey starts with a single step. Be it a workshop or retreat, your choice is the beginning of an exciting new chapter in your yoga journey, a step toward growth, understanding, and peace. Happy journeying, fellow yogi!

Preparing for a Yoga Workshop or Retreat: Tips and Strategies

Venturing into a yoga workshop or retreat is an exciting journey of deepening your practice and self-discovery. Ensuring a rewarding experience requires thoughtful planning and preparation, let's delve into how you can do that.

Map Out Your Intentions

Before you set off, reflect on what you want from the experience. Are you seeking tranquility, a fitness boost, or a deeper connection to your practice? Your intentions will guide you in selecting the right workshop or retreat and setting a personal focus.

Practical Tip: Essential Checklist

- ✓ Research the retreat: Understand the yoga styles offered, daily schedules, and accommodation facilities. Make sure they align with your comfort and preferences.
- ✓ Pack mindfully: Essentials include yoga outfits, mat, meditation cushion, water bottle, healthy snacks, journal, and personal care items. Don't forget a warm shawl for meditation or savasana!
- ✓ Health considerations: Notify the organizers about any dietary restrictions or medical conditions. If needed, consult with your doctor before embarking on the retreat.
- ✓ Mental readiness: Prepare to unplug, be present, and embrace the experience.

Your Preparation Plan Template

Consider this preparation plan as a roadmap guiding you towards a fulfilling retreat experience.

1. **Intentions:** Write down your goals and what you hope to gain from this experience.

    Goal 1:
    _____

    Goal 2:
    _____

Goal 3:
_____

2. **Practical preparations:** Use the provided checklist to ensure you're physically ready.

    Preparation 1:
    _____

    Preparation 2:
    _____

    Preparation 3:
    _____

3. **Mindset:** Jot down ways you can cultivate an open and present mindset during your retreat.

    Goal 1:
    _____

    Goal 2:
    _____

    Goal 3:
    _____

This chapter is the beginning of your retreat adventure. With clear intentions, practical readiness, and an open mind, you're all set to embark on this transformative journey. So, take a deep breath and step forward confidently into your yoga retreat experience, knowing you're well-prepared for the incredible moments of enlightenment that await. Enjoy the journey!

While workshops and retreats offer valuable opportunities to deepen your practice, there is another, more intensive option available if you're seeking an immersive yoga experience: a yoga teacher training program.

The Yoga Teacher Training Experience: An Overview

Embarking on a yoga teacher training journey is like setting sail on an uncharted sea. It's a voyage full of excitement, challenge, transformation, and self-discovery.

Navigating the Seas of Yoga Teacher Training

Imagine stepping into a space dedicated to deepening your understanding of yoga, where each day unravels new layers of this ancient practice, diving deeper into asanas, pranayama, meditation, and yoga philosophy. The training can be rigorous, pushing your physical limits and stretching your mental boundaries. Yet, amid the rigorous asana practices and intense study, you discover a reservoir of inner strength and resilience you never knew you had.

A Personal Anecdote: Maya's Transformation

Remember Maya, the corporate executive we met earlier? Let's revisit her journey, but this time, through the lens of yoga teacher training. Overwhelmed by her high-pressure job, Maya turned to yoga. Her practice became an oasis of calm in the storm of her demanding lifestyle. Inspired to delve deeper, she enrolled in a yoga teacher training program.

During training, Maya encountered challenges she never anticipated – holding asanas for longer periods, learning Sanskrit terms, understanding the subtle energetics of yoga. Despite these challenges, she emerged transformed. Her training became a tool of self-discovery, unearthing her passion for wellness and talent for motivating others. This realization prompted her shift from a corporate executive to a wellness coach, guiding others towards healthier lifestyles.

Reflections: Is Yoga Teacher Training Right for You?

If you're considering a yoga teacher training journey, ponder on these questions: Are you eager to deepen your understanding of yoga beyond what your regular classes offer? Are you ready to step out of your comfort zone and push your boundaries? Do you see yourself sharing the wisdom of yoga with others? Reflecting on these questions might provide the clarity you need.

Remember, yoga teacher training is not solely about becoming a teacher; it's a transformative journey of self-discovery, personal growth, and deepening your practice. It's about stepping onto your mat, day after day, and learning the true essence of yoga: union – of the body, breath, and mind, and ultimately, of the self with the divine. Embark on this journey when your heart feels the call, and when it does, embrace it with openness and curiosity.

Choosing the Right Yoga Teacher Training Program for You

Navigating the vast ocean of yoga teacher training (YTT) programs can be overwhelming. However, with clear intentions and a bit of research, you can find the perfect program to further your yogic journey.

Finding the YTT That Resonates

Choosing the right YTT isn't about finding the most popular or convenient program. It's about finding the program that resonates with your personal goals and values. Are you looking to deepen your personal practice or do you aspire to teach? Are you more drawn towards a specific yoga style or a comprehensive study of many styles?

As you explore different programs, notice how they align with your vision. Do their teaching philosophies resonate with you? Do you connect with the teacher's approach? This personal resonance will be a key ingredient in your growth and satisfaction.

Practical Tips for Making the Right Choice

Curriculum: Examine the curriculum. It should cover essential areas like asanas, pranayama, meditation, anatomy, yoga philosophy, and teaching methodology.

Accreditation: Look for programs accredited by established organizations like Yoga Alliance. This ensures quality and can be important if you plan to teach.

Format: Determine if a residential, non-residential, or online program best suits your schedule and learning preferences.

Teachers: Research the trainers. Their experience, teaching style, and personal philosophy will greatly influence your learning experience.

Alumni Reviews: Read experiences of past students. They provide valuable insights into the program's quality and culture.

Your YTT Decision-Making Worksheet

To simplify your decision-making process, create a worksheet listing all the YTTs you're considering.

- Program Name
- Location
- Duration
- Yoga Styles
- Accreditation
- Cost
- Trainer Profiles
- Curriculum Overview
- Format (residential/non-residential/online)
- Personal Resonance (on a scale of 1-10)

Program Name	location	duration	Yoga Styles	Accreditation	Cost	Trainer Profiles	Curriculum Overview	Format (residential/ commercial / Online)	Personal Resonance (on a scale of 1-10)

Add rows for each program and fill in the details. Pay special attention to the last column – 'Personal Resonance'. Trust your instincts. Sometimes, the right choice isn't the most logical; it's the one that your heart is drawn towards.

Remember, your YTT journey is a personal and transformative one. Choose a program that aligns with your unique path, and the journey will become as fulfilling as the destination.

Maximizing Your Yoga Teacher Training Experience

Embarking on your Yoga Teacher Training (YTT) journey can be a thrilling step into personal growth and transformation. This is your chance to immerse yourself in the essence of yoga. Here are some tips to help you fully engage with this enriching experience.

Prepare Physically, Mentally, and Emotionally

Your YTT journey starts well before the first day of class. It starts with preparation. Deepen your personal practice, read recommended texts, and create a support network to help manage your non-yoga responsibilities. This preparation is not just about getting your body ready, but also your mind and heart. Clear space in your life for this transformative journey.

Engage with an Open Heart and Mind

Approach your YTT with an open heart and mind. Leave your preconceptions at the door. You'll be exposed to new perspectives, techniques, and philosophies. Embrace them. Openness fosters growth.

Practical Tip: The Power of Presence

Embrace the present. The power of YTT isn't solely in the curriculum but also in the living experience. Every practice session, theory class, and group discussion is a treasure trove of valuable insights. By being fully present, you can absorb these lessons and let them permeate your being.

Your YTT Reflection Journal

Given the journaling practices you've developed in the previous chapters, I strongly recommend creating a dedicated YTT Reflection Journal. This can be a sacred space to document your experiences, insights, and emotions during your training.

Prompts to consider:

1. How have my perceptions of yoga changed throughout the training?

2. How have I evolved in my personal practice and teaching skills?
3. What challenges have I encountered, and how did I navigate them?

Remember, YTT isn't just about learning to teach yoga; it's about deepening your relationship with yoga and yourself. It's a transformative journey, one that doesn't end with certification. Enjoy the journey, embrace the lessons, and let the transformative power of yoga work its magic.

The Path of the Yoga Teacher: Exploring Opportunities for Growth and Development

Diving into a yoga retreat or workshop is like exploring uncharted territories of self-discovery. It's a chance to deepen your practice, broaden your knowledge, and potentially transform your life.

Pathways to Growth

Each journey starts with a single step. As a yoga practitioner, that first step may be a class, a book, or even a conversation. Then comes the next step, and the one after that, slowly guiding you along the path of growth and development.

As you plan your own yoga journey, consider workshops and retreats as exciting landmarks. They're opportunities to learn from experts, connect with like-minded souls, and discover new dimensions of your practice.

A Story of Transformation: Naomi's Journey

Let's consider Naomi's story, a high-school teacher who had been practicing yoga for a few years in her local studio. Despite enjoying her routine classes, she felt a growing hunger to delve deeper. She decided to attend a yoga retreat focused on Yin Yoga.

Naomi had read about Yin Yoga and its powerful effects on stress and anxiety, but she'd never practiced it. The retreat turned out to be a profoundly transformative experience. She was immersed in a community of inspiring practitioners and introduced to powerful Yin poses and philosophy.

As she lay in a supported Butterfly pose, surrendering to the pull of gravity, she felt a profound sense of release. This was a transformative moment, opening her up to the profound therapeutic power of Yin.

On returning, Naomi introduced Yin elements into her personal practice, and her students' lives. The retreat had not only deepened her understanding of yoga but also gave her practical tools to better serve her community.

Reflecting on Your Journey

Inspired by Naomi's story, consider how a yoga workshop or retreat might enrich your practice. Take a moment to ponder these reflection questions:

1. What area of yoga would you like to delve deeper into?
2. How might attending a workshop or retreat help you serve your community better?
3. In what ways might this experience facilitate your growth as a yoga practitioner?

As you contemplate these questions, remember that every yoga journey is unique. Yours will be an adventure filled with exciting twists and turns, challenges, and moments of triumph. Prepare yourself with an open heart and mind, and the path of yoga will take you places you've never imagined.

Case Studies: Inspiring Stories from Yoga Teachers and Practitioners

These inspiring stories bear testament to the transformative power of yoga.

Testimonials: Personal Journeys Towards Transformation

Emma and Catherine, both stressed working professionals, found mental clarity and emotional balance through pranayama, showing yoga's calming power amidst chaos.

Take Sophia, a yoga enthusiast. She was struggling with fatigue and weak immunity but witnessed a surge in her health when she explored the Wim Hof Method. Her tale stands as a beacon for those seeking improved wellbeing.

Then we have Michael and Angela, who used the Box Breathing technique to cope with PTSD and academic stress respectively. They saw enhanced emotional regulation and renewed energy, demonstrating yoga's capacity to mend both body and mind.

Reflection on Practice

Reflect on these stories. How might these experiences resonate with your yoga journey?

Continuing the Journey: Deeper Explorations

Next, we revisit Tina, a single mother we met in Chapter 4. She had embraced Kapalabhati and Hatha Yoga earlier. We now find her discovering Ashtanga, demonstrating that yoga can continually challenge and enrich us, regardless of where we are in life.

Ethan too, revisited his practice. Initially, Power Yoga helped him cope with work stress, but he further honed his stress-management toolkit by attending a workshop on yoga and stress relief. His story illustrates how we can delve deeper into our practice, discovering new dimensions of yoga that can better serve us.

Transformation: From Yoga Mats to Life

Our stories do not end on the mat. They extend into our lives, transforming them in myriad ways. Sam, a retired office worker, found a renewed sense of strength and confidence through Chair Yoga, illustrating that yoga can be adapted to serve us at any age.

For Naomi, a high-school teacher, her journey took her to a Yin Yoga retreat. It was there she experienced a deep release and realized the therapeutic power of Yin. She carried this new understanding back to her practice and her classroom, echoing the principle that what we learn on the mat can be used to serve our communities.

In each of these stories, we see how yoga can profoundly transform our lives. As you reflect on these narratives, consider how your own yoga journey might be enriched and deepened.

The Power of Immersion in Yoga

As we draw this chapter to a close, let's reflect on the transformative power of immersion in yoga. The depth, diversity, and richness of yoga are truly unveiled when we dive deep into workshops, retreats, and teacher training programs.

Transformative Tales

Consider Alice's journey as an example. Alice was a school teacher, neck-deep in lesson plans and parent meetings. With a schedule leaving little room for herself, stress was her constant companion. It wasn't until a friend encouraged her to a local yoga workshop that Alice found her escape hatch.

Alice spent her weekends in that safe sanctuary, surrounded by soft music, flickering candles, and the compassionate guidance of her yoga teacher. The workshop opened up a new world of yoga poses, meditation techniques, and deep-dive discussions on yoga philosophy that her usual hour-long classes couldn't offer. Her transformation was nothing short of miraculous. Stress levels dipped, sleep quality improved, and her patience with her students grew tenfold.

Seeing the profound effect of this immersion, Alice sought to deepen her journey, signing up for a yoga retreat and eventually a teacher training program. Today, Alice is not only a school teacher but a passionate yoga instructor, weaving her love for yoga into her school's curriculum, igniting a love for yoga in her students.

Action Plan: Next Steps in Your Yoga Journey

Now, it's your turn to consider your next step. How can you deepen your own practice? Maybe a local workshop has caught your eye, or perhaps a week-long retreat in a serene mountain hideaway? Or is it time to consider a teacher training program, sharing the gift of yoga with others?

Here's an interactive action plan template:

Yoga Workshop:

1. *What type of workshop intrigues you? (i.e., focus on asanas, meditation, pranayama, etc.)*

   _____
   _____

2. *Timeline: When do you plan to attend it?*

   _____
   _____
   _____

Yoga Retreat

1. *What kind of retreat do you desire? (i.e., local, international, thematic, etc.)*

   _____

   _____

   _____

2. *Timeline: When can you take out time for this retreat?*

   _____

   _____

   _____

Teacher Training Program

1. *What's driving you towards becoming a yoga teacher?*

   _____

   _____

   _____

2. *Timeline: When do you plan to start your training?*

   _____

   _____

   _____

In this chapter, we have delved deep into maximizing your Yoga Teacher Training (YTT) experience and explored various opportunities for growth and development through yoga workshops, retreats, and teacher training programs. We've learned the transformative power of immersion in yoga through inspiring stories and personal journeys towards transformation. Let's carry forward this knowledge as we continue our yoga journey.

Creating Closure and Looking Ahead

Just like Alice, you too can transform your life with yoga immersion. Reflect on this: How can immersing in yoga through workshops, retreats, or teacher training shape your practice? What transformations are you seeking, and how can yoga help you achieve them?

Challenge yourself to deepen your yoga practice this week. Perhaps you can attend a yoga workshop in your local community, try a Yin yoga class for stress relief, or even explore a new breathing technique like the Box Breathing method we've discussed. This is your journey, and you have the power to shape it. Remember, every journey begins with a single step.

Additionally, start laying the groundwork for the next step in your yoga journey - building your yoga community. Try attending a yoga event in your local community or start a conversation with a fellow yoga practitioner after your next class.

With anticipation, let's look to our next chapter, where we delve into the power of community in your yoga journey. We'll explore how finding your 'tribe' can bolster your practice, offering support, motivation, and a sense of belonging. See you in 'Chapter 19: Building a Supportive Yoga Community.

Remember, 'Yoga is a light, which once lit, will never dim. The better your practice, the brighter the flame.' - B.K.S. Iyengar. Let this light guide you on your journey towards transformation.

19

Building a Supportive Yoga Community

Welcome, dear reader, to the next chapter in your yoga journey. After exploring the transformative power of immersion in yoga through workshops, retreats, and teacher training, we're now turning our focus towards a crucial aspect of your practice: community. Just as our last chapter's closing reflections encouraged you to delve deeper into your practice, our journey forward will be similarly rewarding, allowing us to discover how nurturing a supportive yoga community can enrich your experience and personal growth.

The Power of Community in Yoga

A supportive yoga community, or 'sangha' as it's often called in yogic tradition, is a powerful force. It's a space where we share our experiences, our triumphs, our challenges, and our discoveries. It offers a sense of belonging, mutual encouragement, and inspiration. Practicing in a community allows us to learn from others, drawing from their insights and experiences. It's a comforting echo reminding us that we are not alone on this path. In fact, we're part of a global network of souls connected by the common thread of yoga.

Where Do You Stand in Your Yoga Community?

Before we delve deeper, let's take a moment to understand your current standing in your yoga community. Take this short quiz to evaluate your level of involvement.

1. How often do you engage in yoga activities with others? (weekly classes, workshops, retreats)
2. Do you share and discuss your yoga experiences with others?

3. How often do you participate in yoga events in your local area?
4. Have you ever volunteered or offered your services in a yoga-related activity?
5. Do you actively seek out opportunities to connect with other yoga practitioners?

The goal of this quiz is not to measure or judge, but to inspire self-reflection. Recognizing where we stand is the first step in charting a course towards where we want to be.

With this chapter's focus on 'Building a Supportive Yoga Community', we are stepping into a space filled with warmth, connection, and shared growth. As we dive deeper, we'll uncover strategies to find your tribe, nurture connections, and bolster your practice through community engagement. Remember, every step in your journey is important, including the people you walk with along the way.

Yoga is a light, illuminating our path, while community is the force that propels us forward. Let's explore how to harness this collective energy in our next section: 'Finding Your Tribe: Nurturing Your Yoga Community.' We'll delve into practical ways to build your yoga community, and continue to fan the flame of your yoga journey.

"Individually, we are one drop. Together, we are an ocean." - Ryunosuke Satoro. Let's dive into this ocean of shared experience, ready to navigate the currents of communal practice.

The Importance of Community in Your Yoga Journey

Embarking on a journey into yoga can often seem like a solitary experience; however, finding your tribe and becoming a part of a yoga community can be as enriching as the practice itself.

A Shared Experience

A community brings a shared sense of purpose and mutual understanding. It's where stories intertwine, and personal growth blooms from collective experience. Your fellow practitioners can encourage you when you feel stuck, cheer you on as you break through your limits, and share in the joy of your victories. A yoga community can offer a nurturing space for transformation and a platform for growth.

Naomi's Journey: The Power of a Yoga Community

To truly understand the impact of a supportive yoga community, let's revisit Naomi's journey. Naomi, a high-school teacher, delved deeper into her yoga practice at a Yin Yoga retreat. This retreat was more than just a deep dive into Yin poses and philosophy. It was a collective journey of like-minded individuals, sharing experiences, insights, and moments of revelation. Naomi didn't just return with a deeper understanding of yoga; she brought back a sense of belonging that came from being part of a community.

Back home, Naomi's enriched practice had a ripple effect. She started incorporating Yin elements into her teaching, not just impacting her students' physical wellness but also creating a microcosm of a supportive yoga community right within her classroom. This is the transformative power of a yoga community - it doesn't just change you; it enables you to bring about change in the lives of others.

Your Role in Your Yoga Community

Now, it's time for you to reflect on your role in your yoga community. Consider the following questions:

1. How active are you in your yoga community?
2. Do you share your experiences and insights with others?
3. How do you contribute to the growth and enrichment of your yoga community?
4. How has your yoga community influenced your practice and personal growth?

As we journey ahead in this chapter, we'll delve deeper into ways you can nurture your connections within your yoga community and how it can, in turn, bolster your practice. Remember, a strong community can create a vibrant environment for collective and personal growth, adding a new dimension to your yoga journey.

Finding and Connecting with Like-Minded Individuals

Embarking on your yoga journey can be exciting and transformative, but it's even more enriching when shared with like-minded individuals. As we saw with Naomi's story in the previous section, a supportive community can amplify personal growth and extend the impact of yoga beyond the mat. So, how do you find and connect with your tribe within the yoga community?

Identifying Your Tribe

Firstly, identifying your tribe starts with understanding your personal yoga journey. What are your interests and goals in practicing yoga? Are you looking for physical fitness, stress relief, or spiritual growth? Reflecting on these aspects can guide you towards individuals or groups with similar objectives.

Practical Tip: Yoga Community Networking

Once you've defined what you're looking for, it's time to explore! Attend different yoga classes, workshops, and retreats. Participate in online yoga forums or join social media groups dedicated to yoga. These are all great places to meet like-minded individuals.

Be open and genuine in your interactions. Share your experiences, ask questions, and show interest in other people's journeys. Remember, networking isn't just about finding people; it's about forging meaningful connections.

Alice's Journey: The Impact of Networking

Let's look back at Alice's story for inspiration. Overwhelmed by work stress, Alice found solace in a local yoga workshop. This initial step led her to a broader yoga community where she discovered a shared passion for yoga's transformative power. Inspired by her personal transformation, she decided to become a yoga instructor, integrating yoga into her school's curriculum. Alice's story beautifully illustrates how connecting with the right individuals can catalyze significant change.

Your Yoga Community Networking Plan

Now, it's time to plan your own journey of connection. Here's a simple networking plan template:

> **Objectives:** Define what you are hoping to achieve by connecting with like-minded individuals.
>
> **Opportunities:** Identify places or platforms where you might meet these individuals.
>
> **Actions:** Outline specific actions you'll take to engage with these individuals or groups.

Reflection: Set a date to review your progress and reflect on your experiences.

YOGA COMMUNITY NETWORKING PLAN

OBJECTIVES

[Define what you are hoping to achieve by connecting with like-minded individuals.]

_____
_____
_____

OPPORTUNITIES

[Identify places or platforms where you might meet these individuals.]

_____
_____
_____

ACTIONS

[Outline specific actions you'll take to engage with these individuals or groups.]

_____
_____
_____

REFLECTION

[Set a date to review your progress and reflect on your experiences.]

_____

Building meaningful connections takes time and effort, but the rewards are immeasurable. A strong yoga community can provide support, encouragement, and shared joy along your yoga journey. So take the first step, reach out, and let your yoga practice be enriched by the power of a like-minded community.

Creating a Safe and Inclusive Space for Yoga Practice

Yoga is for everyone. One of the most empowering aspects of the practice is its inclusivity. It's about connecting with your inner self, and in the process, encouraging others to do the same. A safe and inclusive space is integral to fostering this connection.

Why a Safe and Inclusive Yoga Space Matters

Creating a space where everyone feels welcomed and respected enhances the overall yoga experience. It fosters a sense of belonging, strengthens community bonds, and deepens individual and collective practice. It helps break down barriers, allowing every participant to feel comfortable sharing their journey and growing in their practice.

Practical Tips: Building an Inclusive Yoga Space

Here's a checklist to consider:

- ✓ **Accessibility:** Is your space physically accessible to all, including those with mobility limitations?
- ✓ **Respect for diversity:** Are you acknowledging and respecting all ethnicities, genders, ages, sizes, and abilities in your yoga space?
- ✓ **Safe practice:** Are you ensuring that safety measures are in place, including modifying poses to cater to all levels of fitness and health?
- ✓ **Open communication:** Do you encourage open dialogue and feedback about participants' comfort and well-being?

Reflecting on Your Yoga Space

Ask yourself these questions:

1. What measures have I taken to ensure my yoga space is inclusive?
2. How do I make my yoga space physically and emotionally safe for everyone?
3. How could I improve the inclusivity and safety of my yoga space?

Your answers can guide you towards creating a more welcoming environment, where everyone can explore their yoga journey in a supportive, nurturing atmosphere.

Tips for Nurturing and Growing Your Yoga Community

The heart of yoga lies in community—a supportive network that breathes, stretches, and evolves together. Nurturing this community is like tending a garden, requiring patience, love, and care. Let's delve into how you can sow the seeds of connection, cultivate relationships, and watch your yoga community bloom.

The Power of Community in Yoga

Community is an often-overlooked aspect of yoga. It's the collective energy of your fellow yogis that uplifts you when you stumble, cheers you on as you conquer a challenging pose, and supports you through the highs and lows of your yoga journey. A thriving yoga community can transform individual practice into a collective experience, amplifying the benefits of yoga and fostering a sense of shared accomplishment.

Practical Tips: Cultivating Your Yoga Community

Here are some tips to foster engagement and growth in your yoga community:

1. **Host special events:** Workshops, retreats, and guest lectures offer valuable opportunities for learning and connection. Make these events interactive and fun, encouraging everyone to participate.
2. **Promote inclusivity:** Welcome all ages, backgrounds, and abilities. Celebrate diversity and create an environment where everyone feels seen and appreciated.
3. **Foster open communication:** Encourage dialogue, listen to feedback, and involve your community in decision-making. This promotes a sense of ownership and strengthens community bonds.
4. **Prioritize community wellness:** Integrate mindfulness practices, wellness tips, and self-care reminders into your teachings. Show your community that their well-being matters to you.
5. **Create online spaces:** Establish an online forum where your community can share thoughts, ideas, and experiences. This keeps the connection strong even when physical meetings are not possible.

6. **Collaborate with local businesses:** Partnering with local businesses can lead to mutual promotion, cross-over events, and unique experiences that add value to your community.

Your Community Development Plan

Having a community development plan helps in guiding your actions and decisions. Here's a simple template:

- **Objectives:** What are your goals for the community? How do you see it evolving?
- **Opportunities:** Identify the opportunities for community-building. Are there events, collaborations, or initiatives you can leverage?
- **Actions:** List the specific steps you'll take to achieve your objectives and seize your opportunities.
- **Review and Reflect:** Set a date to review your progress and reflect on what's working and what needs to be improved.

Cultivating a thriving yoga community is a journey of connection and growth. By nurturing your community with intention and care, you're not only enhancing your own yoga experience but also enriching the journey of every member of your community. Remember, every tree in a forest contributes to the health of the whole, and every yogi in your community contributes to the collective energy. So, let's roll out our mats, breathe together, and let our community grow in strength and spirit.

Incorporating Yoga Service and Outreach Programs

Service and outreach are fundamental principles of yoga that extend beyond the boundaries of the mat, fostering inclusivity, connection, and mutual growth. By incorporating these programs into our yoga practice, we can create a ripple effect of positivity and transformation within our communities.

The Essence of Yoga Service and Outreach

Yoga service and outreach programs are initiatives designed to extend the benefits of yoga to those who may not have easy access to it due to social, economic, or physical barriers. They aim to create inclusive spaces where everyone can benefit from yoga, regardless of their circumstances. Such programs often target underserved populations, addressing unique needs and fostering a sense of community, self-worth, and empowerment.

Personal Story: Alice's Journey into Yoga Service and Outreach

Let's journey back to Alice's transformative encounter with yoga. Remember Alice? The school teacher who initially sought solace in yoga from work stress and ended up integrating it into her school's curriculum. But her yoga journey didn't stop there.

Alice recognized that yoga could reach beyond her school to serve her wider community. She developed an outreach program, taking yoga to local community centers and senior living homes. These sessions were often the highlight of her week, with the laughter, shared stories, and glowing faces of participants illuminating the power of yoga to bring joy and connection. Alice witnessed yoga's transformative effect on her students—easing anxiety, enhancing mobility, and fostering a sense of community among individuals who had often felt isolated or excluded.

Reflecting on Your Yoga Service Journey

1. **Identify:** Can you identify a group within your community that could benefit from yoga but currently lacks access or resources?
2. **Explore:** What barriers might prevent this group from experiencing the benefits of yoga? How could you address these barriers?
3. **Envision:** How could a yoga service or outreach program enhance the well-being of this group and the wider community?
4. **Plan:** What steps could you take to initiate a yoga service or outreach program?

Alice's story illustrates how yoga service and outreach programs can bring the holistic benefits of yoga to those who may otherwise miss out. By considering your potential role in these initiatives, you can contribute to expanding the reach of yoga and fostering a truly inclusive and supportive yoga community. The beauty of yoga service lies in its reciprocity - as you extend the reach of yoga, you'll find your own practice enriched by the diversity and shared experiences of your expanding yoga community.

Online Yoga Communities: Benefits and Strategies for Connection

The beauty of yoga is its ability to adapt and flourish in diverse environments. With the rise of digital platforms, the global yoga community has embraced the virtual world, connecting practitioners from all walks of life. Online yoga communities are flourishing, offering a myriad of benefits and opportunities for connection.

Benefits of Online Yoga Communities

Online yoga communities transcend geographical boundaries, offering a diverse, inclusive space for individuals to practice, learn, and grow. These digital platforms provide access to a wide range of resources, from tutorials to live classes, and forums for discussion and exchange. They foster a sense of global community, connection, and shared journey, bolstering your practice with collective wisdom and support.

Practical Tip: Navigating Online Yoga Communities

Successfully navigating online yoga communities requires an open mind and an eagerness to engage. Start by exploring different platforms and groups to find those that resonate with your goals and values. Participate in discussions, attend live classes, and be open to the diverse perspectives you'll encounter.

Remember, everyone in the online yoga community is on their unique yoga journey. Be respectful and supportive of other members, understanding that we are all learning and growing together. Encourage and inspire others with your journey, and let their journeys inspire you.

Creating a Robust Online Yoga Community Presence

Crafting a robust online yoga presence can be a fulfilling and rewarding experience. Here's a step-by-step guide to help you along the way:

> **Define Your Intentions:** Identify what you want from your online yoga community. Are you seeking inspiration, companionship, or support in your yoga journey?

Choose Your Platforms: Research various online yoga platforms and choose those that align with your intentions.

Engage Authentically: Authenticity fosters genuine connections. Share your experiences, ask questions, and participate in discussions genuinely.

Be Consistent: Consistent participation keeps you connected and active within the community.

Offer Support: Provide encouragement and support to other members. Your words can be a source of inspiration and motivation for others.

As we journey together in our yoga practices, online communities provide a global platform for connection, sharing, and growth. So, unroll your digital yoga mat, step into the virtual yoga world, and enrich your practice with the collective wisdom of yogis worldwide. Remember, the essence of yoga lies not just in perfecting asanas but in connecting with ourselves and others, nurturing a global community of peace, unity, and shared growth.

Interactive Exercise: Building Your Personal Yoga Support Network

Crafting a supportive yoga network is integral to nurturing your practice, and this interactive exercise is designed to guide you through this process. It's about fostering connections, sharing experiences, and creating a collective energy that fuels your yoga journey.

Practical Tip: Steps to Build a Supportive Yoga Network

1. **Identify Your Needs:** Determine what you need from your network. Support? Inspiration? A practice buddy?
2. **Seek Like-Minded Yogis:** Connect with individuals who share similar goals and values.
3. **Engage Actively:** Participate in yoga classes, workshops, and online communities to meet and interact with fellow practitioners.

4. **Foster Relationships:** Building a network is about fostering relationships. Be open, supportive, and engage authentically with your yoga community.

Your Networking Action Plan

Ready to craft your personal yoga support network? Here's a simple template to guide you:

- **My Yoga Support Network Goals:** What do you hope to gain from your yoga network?
- **Potential Connections:** List people you know who practice yoga or are interested in starting.
- **Outreach Strategy:** How will you reach out to potential connections? Consider social media, yoga classes, and workshops.
- **Engagement Plan:** Detail how you plan to actively participate in your network.

Your yoga journey is not just a personal endeavor, but a collective experience. As you connect with others, share your journey, and draw inspiration from theirs, you'll discover the true essence of yoga. Remember, each connection you foster enriches not just your practice, but also that of the entire yoga community. The bond of a yoga network transcends the confines of the yoga mat, creating a shared path of wellness, growth, and unity. So, let's start crafting your personal yoga support network today!

Case Studies: Inspiring Stories of Yoga Communities and Connections

Diving into real-life tales of transformation, we'll witness the undeniable power of yoga communities and connections. These stories are a testament to yoga's potential to reshape lives, reaffirming our belief in its universal relevance.

Dylan's Journey: Discovering the Power of Collective Healing

Dylan was a decorated military veteran grappling with the silent war of PTSD. Feeling isolated and misunderstood, he discovered an online community of veterans practicing yoga as a healing journey. The community was an oasis of shared experiences, empathy, and encouragement. Dylan found a renewed sense of purpose, using yoga as a tool for self-healing and connecting with other veterans on a similar journey.

Amanda's Tale: Building a Global Yoga Family

Amanda was an enthusiastic yoga practitioner from a small Midwestern town, eager to connect with like-minded yogis. She started an Instagram page, sharing her yoga journey and insights. Her genuine enthusiasm resonated with many, and she soon had followers from around the world. Amanda's page wasn't just about asanas or meditation techniques; it became a space for yogis to connect, share, and learn from each other, essentially creating a global yoga family.

Reflection and Projection

Consider Dylan's and Amanda's experiences and ask yourself these reflection questions:

1. How could belonging to a supportive yoga community enhance your own yoga journey?
2. Could sharing your yoga journey, like Amanda, create meaningful connections and inspire others?
3. Do Dylan's experiences reveal any personal obstacles that a yoga community could help you overcome?

Allow these stories to inspire you, reminding you of the powerful connection between yoga and community. They are more than just individual experiences; they represent the collective potential of a yoga community to heal, inspire, and connect.

The Power of Community in Yoga

Reflecting on the Power of Community

Our journey through the yoga practice takes different shapes and forms, but one aspect that remains undeniably powerful is the community it fosters. Reflecting on this chapter, we've discovered how the yoga community can uplift us, challenge us, and transform us. It deepens our understanding of ourselves and our practice, fostering a sense of belonging that nurtures our spirit as we traverse our yoga path.

Personal Story: Transformation through Community

Consider Rachel, a dedicated yoga practitioner. She was a lone yogi for years, practicing at home due to shyness. One day, she stepped out of her comfort zone and joined a local yoga studio. The supportive community she found there was transformative. Rachel not only grew in her practice, but she also discovered a resilience she hadn't recognized in herself before. She became more open, more confident, and found a new sense of camaraderie that was profoundly healing.

Action Plan: Building Your Yoga Community

Now it's your turn. Are you ready to connect with your yoga community or maybe even start your own? Use the template provided to draft your action plan. Outline how you'll reach out to fellow practitioners, participate in community events, or even lead a class yourself. Start small and allow this plan to evolve as you grow in your journey.

YOGA COMMUNITY ACTION PLANGoal Setting:

Goal Setting:

     a. Long-Term Goal: What is your ultimate goal with your yoga community? Do you want to join an existing one, start your own, or perhaps deepen your involvement in your current one?

     _____
     _____
     _____

     b. Short-Term Goals: Break down your long-term goal into smaller, more manageable steps. What can you achieve in a month? Three months? Six months?

     _____
     _____
     _____

Resources:

a. Existing Resources: What resources do you already have that can help you achieve your goals? This could be yoga mats, a suitable space for practice, or a yoga teacher certification.

_____
_____
_____

b. Needed Resources: What resources do you need to acquire to move forward with your goals? How will you obtain these?

_____
_____
_____

Action Steps:

a. Step One: What is the first step you will take to achieve your short-term goal? This could be researching local yoga communities, reaching out to potential members for your own community, or taking a class to deepen your involvement.

_____
_____
_____

b. Step Two: What will be your next step? And the one after that?

_____
_____
_____

Continue this process for each step toward your short-term and long-term goals.

Timeline:

    a. Start Date: When will you begin working towards your goals?

_____

_____

_____

    b. Milestone Dates: What are the target dates for your short-term goals?

_____

_____

_____

    c. End Date: When do you hope to achieve your long-term goal?

_____

_____

_____

Notes & Reflections:

    This space is for you to jot down any thoughts, feelings, or observations as you work through your action plan. Reflecting on your journey can provide invaluable insights and keep you motivated.

_____

_____

_____

Remember, this action plan is a living document. You can change it, update it, and adjust it as you continue your journey. Good luck, and enjoy building and nurturing your yoga community!

Your Journey Ahead

Reflect on your yoga journey so far. How has the community aspect influenced you? How can you nurture this moving forward? Embrace this moment of reflection and consider your next steps. Remember, your journey is unique, and the way you engage with your yoga community should resonate with your spirit.

Our journey doesn't stop here. As we close this chapter, take a moment to celebrate your achievements and contemplate your yoga future. You've armed yourself with knowledge and strategies, and now you're ready to take on new challenges.

Get excited for our next chapter, "Celebrating Your Inner Light: A Journey of Self-Discovery and Transformation." There, we'll delve into the deeper aspects of personal growth, exploring the ways yoga can illuminate the inner light within you. Keep this sense of community in your heart as we continue, for it is a significant part of your yoga journey. Together, we will delve deeper, stretch further, and continue to grow. Namaste.

20

Celebrating Your Inner Light: A Journey of Self-Discovery and Transformation

Welcome, dear yogis, to the penultimate chapter of our shared journey, where we will explore the beautiful process of self-discovery and transformation. By now, you have forged meaningful connections with your yoga community, honed your physical practice, and begun to truly comprehend the power of yoga in your life. Now, it's time to turn our gaze inward and celebrate your inner light.

Discovering Your Inner Light

Yoga, at its core, is a journey of self-discovery. Every asana, every breath, and every moment of mindfulness is a step closer to your true self, that spark of divinity that resides within you. In this chapter, we will explore how yoga can help you discover and nurture this inner light.

Transformative Power of Yoga

The practice of yoga transcends physical movement—it has the power to transform us from within. This transformation is not a destination but a continual journey, a process of becoming. Here, we'll look at how your practice has initiated this transformative journey and how to continue fostering it.

Reflecting on Your Yoga Journey

As we embark on this chapter, take a moment to reflect on your journey so far. How has yoga transformed you? How have you seen your inner light manifest in your daily life? To aid in this reflection, you'll find a simple, yet insightful quiz at the end of this section. It's designed to help you pause and ponder on your growth, shedding light on the areas you've blossomed in and those that might need a bit more nurturing.

The Ongoing Journey

While we are nearing the end of this book, remember that your yoga journey is a lifelong expedition of growth, discovery, and transformation. As we approach the final pages, let's take the time to honor the progress you've made, while also acknowledging the beautiful journey that lies ahead.

In the coming pages, we'll dive deeper into each of these topics, guided by the collective wisdom of our yoga community and fueled by your personal experiences. Let's embark on this path of self-discovery and transformation, celebrating the brilliant inner light that makes you, uniquely you. Namaste

Reflecting on Your Personal Yoga Journey

Life is a journey of countless stories woven together with our triumphs, failures, discoveries, and transformations. One such precious tale is your personal yoga journey - a path adorned with self-discovery, healing, resilience, and growth. Let's explore this trail, reflecting on the insights gained, and celebrate your transformation.

Understanding Your Journey

Reflecting on your journey means acknowledging the path you've taken and the transformations you've undergone. From the moment you first rolled out your mat, the challenges you've encountered, the breakthroughs experienced, the resilience developed, and the harmony found - these are all integral parts of your personal yoga narrative.

Consider Tina's journey, introduced in Chapter 4. From a single mother overwhelmed by life's demands to a woman finding balance through Hatha Yoga and later exploring the challenge of Ashtanga. This story echoes your own, in unique ways, of course. The evolution of your practice, the deepening of your self-understanding, and the embodiment of yoga's principles are your shared chapters.

Insights from a Seasoned Yogi: My Yoga Odyssey

Let's consider my personal story as a seasoned yogi. Like a sapling, I started my practice in shaky soil, questioning every pose, every breath. Over time, I found my roots deepening into the rich soil of self-discovery, flexibility, strength, and tranquility. I learned to respect my body's boundaries and honor its capabilities. Years later, I am not merely a tree standing tall, but a forest thriving with life. This journey was not just about mastering poses but understanding myself and my inner universe.

Interactive Reflection: Document Your Journey

So, where do you find yourself in your yoga journey? What challenges have you overcome? What transformations have you experienced?

Here are some reflection questions to guide your thoughts:

1. What initially drew you to yoga? How has that motivation evolved?
2. How has your physical, mental, or emotional health changed since you began practicing?
3. What was a significant milestone or turning point in your journey?

Take some time to journal your thoughts, and don't rush this process. Allow your experiences, thoughts, and feelings to flow onto the paper, just as you would flow through your poses on the mat.

Personal Yoga Journey: A Lifelong Odyssey

Your yoga journey is more than a sequence of poses; it's a holistic process of self-discovery, self-love, resilience, and continuous growth. Remember, the beauty of your journey lies not just in the destination but also in the path itself. In the words of Naomi, who discovered a new depth in her practice at a Yin Yoga retreat, "Every asana, every breath is a step towards self-discovery. It's a journey within a journey, and each step is transformative in its own beautiful way."

Remember, your yoga journey is a lifelong odyssey. Embrace the transformation, cherish the growth, and remember to reflect and celebrate your progress. Here's to the many beautiful chapters that await you on your personal yoga journey!

Embracing and Celebrating Your Inner Light

Unveiling Your Inner Light: The Heart of Yoga

At the core of every one of us lies a profound source of wisdom, strength, and radiance – our inner light. In yoga philosophy, this light represents our true self, the unchanging essence beneath the fluctuations of mind and body. It's a concept deeply interwoven in the fabric of yoga, an eternal spark of divine consciousness residing within each of us.

This inner light is ever-present, even amidst the storms of life. Yet, we often forget its existence, consumed by external circumstances and distractions. Embracing and celebrating your inner light means acknowledging its presence, kindling its radiance, and letting it guide your yoga journey and life.

Practical Guide: Igniting Your Inner Light

Recognizing and celebrating your inner light is a deeply personal journey. It requires self-reflection, mindfulness, and commitment. But rest assured, the rewards are boundless.

> **1. Dedicate** Your Practice: In your yoga practice, consciously dedicate each session to honoring your inner light. As you move through your asanas, visualize the flow of energy stimulating your inner radiance.

> **2. Meditate:** Meditation allows for a deeper connection with your inner self. Practice meditations focused on self-love and acceptance, lighting the path towards your inner spark.

> **3. Live Mindfully:** Extend your yoga practice beyond the mat. Embody the principles of yoga in your daily life. Express gratitude, practice kindness, and be present in each moment.

> **4. Seek Inspiration:** Consider stories from fellow yogis who've harnessed their inner light. Sarah, for instance, discovered her innate talent for painting through mindful yoga, radiating her inner light through her art.

> **5. Celebrate:** Celebrate your journey, acknowledging your progress. Each step you take towards embracing your inner light is a victory worth celebrating.

Interactive Reflection: Illuminate Your Path

To evaluate how you embrace and celebrate your inner light, here's a self-reflection exercise. Ask yourself:

1. How do you perceive your inner light? What does it represent for you?
2. In what moments do you feel your inner light shining the brightest?
3. How do you nurture your inner light through yoga and in your daily life?
4. What obstacles do you face in acknowledging and celebrating your inner light?
5. How can you better honor and express your inner light?

Note down your thoughts and revisit them periodically. They will serve as precious milestones on your journey towards embracing and celebrating your inner light.

Embracing Your Inner Light: A Celebration of Self

Your inner light is your eternal companion on your yoga journey and in life. To embrace it is to honor your truth, your essence. To celebrate it is to radiate your unique brilliance, echoing Mark's journey of discovering his creative side through yoga and letting it shine. Your inner light is your guiding star, leading you towards self-discovery, fulfillment, and a harmonious dance with life. Embrace it, celebrate it, and let your inner light shine!

The Importance of Patience and Perseverance on Your Yoga Path

Navigating the Yoga Path: Patience and Perseverance

Embarking on the journey of yoga is akin to setting sail on a vast ocean of self-discovery. It's an exciting voyage, full of ebbs and flows, calm stretches, and stormy waters. Two virtues become your faithful navigators in this journey – patience and perseverance.

Patience is the gentle wind that propels your sailboat, allowing you to flow with the current of your personal growth, without striving to rush or resist. Perseverance, on the other hand, is your steady rudder, guiding you through challenging waters and keeping you aligned with your true north.

In the yoga asana practice and life alike, patience and perseverance are crucial. They allow us to remain committed during challenging poses, maintain calm when progress seems slow, and keep going despite hurdles, much like James's journey towards recovery and enhanced performance through diaphragmatic breathing, showing patience with his injury and perseverance in his practice.

Practical Steps: Cultivating Patience and Perseverance

Harnessing patience and perseverance takes mindful effort. Here are some strategies to guide you:

1. Set Intentional Goals: Define what you aim to achieve in your yoga practice. Remember, progress in yoga is not just about nailing a challenging pose; it's also about developing mindfulness, compassion, and resilience.

2. Embrace the Process: Celebrate the journey rather than just the outcome. Each step of your yoga practice is an opportunity for learning and growth.

3. Practice Mindfulness: Stay present in each moment, whether it's during a challenging asana or a day of struggle. Acknowledge your feelings without judgment.

4. Build Resilience: When you face obstacles, remind yourself of your inner strength. Recall instances when you've overcome challenges, drawing inspiration from those moments.

Interactive Reflection: Assessing Patience and Perseverance

Reflecting on your personal journey can offer valuable insights into your relationship with patience and perseverance. Consider these questions:

1. How patient are you with your progress in your yoga practice and in life?
2. In moments of struggle, how do you exercise perseverance?
3. Are there times when you could have shown more patience or perseverance? How would that have changed the situation?

4. What are some ways you can cultivate more patience and perseverance in your yoga practice and daily life?

Documenting your reflections can be a potent tool for personal growth, encouraging mindfulness and intentional living.

Patience and Perseverance: The Anchors of Your Yoga Journey

Embodying patience and perseverance illuminates your yoga path, turning every challenge into an opportunity for growth and every setback into a springboard for resilience. Like in Tina's story, where her patience with her demanding life circumstances and perseverance in her practice led her to a more balanced and enriched life. Remember, every wave you sail through, every storm you weather, brings you closer to your true self. In your yoga journey and life, patience and perseverance are your most trusted companions. Embrace them, and watch your inner strength unfold.

The Ongoing Journey of Personal Growth and Transformation

The Unfolding Journey: Personal Growth and Transformation

Life is a magnificent journey of evolution, a continual dance of growth and transformation. In the world of yoga, this dance becomes a vividly tangible experience, as you begin to connect deeper with your body, mind, and spirit, much like a lotus unfolding its petals.

Glimpses of Transformation: Rachel's Story

Remember Rachel, our lone yogi turned community nurturer? Her tale is an inspiring testament to the transformative power of yoga. For years, Rachel practiced yoga alone, cocooned within the safe confines of her home, shying away from the gaze of others. The decision to step outside her comfort zone and join a local studio sparked a shift in her life and her yoga journey.

The warm embrace of the yoga community became the sunshine that encouraged Rachel's lotus to blossom. Her yoga practice deepened, but even more importantly, her self-perception underwent a sea-change. The shy, solitary practitioner morphed into a confident community member, radiating resilience and camaraderie. She was no longer just a yogi; she was part of a tribe, a collective journey towards well-being.

Goal-Setting for Transformation

To facilitate your personal journey of transformation, setting clear, achievable goals is essential. Below is an interactive exercise to guide you:

1. **Define Your Vision:** What does your ideal yoga journey look like? Do you see yourself mastering a challenging asana or deepening your meditative practices?
2. **Set Specific Goals:** Break down your vision into smaller, specific goals. Make sure they are realistic and within your capabilities.
3. **Develop an Action Plan:** Outline a step-by-step path to reach each goal. This could involve attending more classes, dedicating more time to practice, or seeking guidance from a mentor.
4. **Monitor Your Progress:** Regularly assess your progress. Celebrate your victories, no matter how small, and reassess your strategies if necessary.
5. **Reflect and Revise:** As you evolve, your goals might change. Regular reflection ensures your goals align with your current aspirations and capabilities.

Your journey of personal growth and transformation is a lifelong adventure, one that yoga can illuminate in unexpected ways. Just as Rachel transformed from a shy, solitary practitioner into a confident, community-oriented yogi, so too can you blossom in your unique way. And remember, this transformation isn't a solitary process; it's nurtured by the collective energy of the yoga community, where every individual journey contributes to the shared tapestry of growth and transformation. As you progress in your yoga path, may you bloom like the lotus, reaching for the light of your fullest potential.

Recognizing the Impact of Your Inner Light on Others

Each one of us holds an inner light, an inherent radiance that can profoundly affect the world around us. This light, when nurtured, becomes a beacon of positivity that touches everyone we come in contact with. Just as a candle can ignite a thousand others without losing its flame, so can your inner light illuminate the paths of others.

The Illuminating Ripple Effect

Look at the stories we've explored together: Rachel's transformation through her local yoga community, Tina's balancing journey through Hatha Yoga, or Lisa, the violinist who shared her talent, enriching the lives of many. Each of them had a light within that when acknowledged, brought change not only to their lives but also had a ripple effect on their surroundings.

Personal Story: Naomi's Illuminating Journey

Take Naomi, the high-school teacher. When she delved deeper into Yin Yoga, it wasn't just about her personal growth. She took what she learned and implemented it in her teachings. Her students, and the wider school community, benefited from the enhanced knowledge and practice she brought. This led to a more mindful, relaxed atmosphere that positively impacted student's performance and overall wellbeing. A testament to the radiance of Naomi's inner light.

Naomi's journey demonstrates that our inner light does not merely exist to benefit us alone. It is a gift to be shared, a positive force that has the potential to extend beyond our immediate sphere and positively impact our community.

Reflecting on Your Inner Light

Reflecting on our stories, consider your own practice and personal journey.

1. How has your inner light grown and developed through your yoga journey?
2. Can you identify specific moments where your inner light has positively impacted those around you?
3. How can you continue to nurture your inner light and use it to bring positivity to your community?

Remember, like Naomi and others, your journey doesn't exist in isolation. Every step you take, every breath you make, sends ripples into the world. As you continue to shine your inner light, you contribute to the collective light that illuminates our world.

Interactive Exercise: Crafting Your Personal Yoga Mission Statement

A personal yoga mission statement is your compass, guiding your journey towards balance, harmony, and self-discovery. By crafting a mission statement, you define your yoga path, understanding what you seek from the practice, and how it aligns with your life goals.

Guided Steps to Your Mission Statement

- **Step 1: Identify Your Yoga Values**

    What does yoga mean to you? Is it a tool for relaxation, a path to spiritual growth, a way to improve physical fitness, or all of the above? List these values down.

- **Step 2: Visualize Your Ideal Yoga Self**

    How do you see yourself in the future through the lens of yoga? Visualize the best version of your yoga self, jotting down the qualities and habits that this version of you embodies.

- **Step 3: Define Your Goals**

    What are your goals in relation to your yoga practice? These could be physical (like mastering a particular pose), mental (such as developing mindfulness), or spiritual (like cultivating inner peace).

- **Step 4: Craft Your Statement**

    Combine your values, visualizations, and goals into a coherent, inspiring mission statement. It should reflect who you are, who you aspire to be, and how yoga can help you get there.

Template for Your Yoga Mission Statement

I, (Your Name), commit to cultivating a yoga practice grounded in (Your Values). Through yoga, I aspire to become (Your Ideal Yoga Self), striving towards (Your Goals). I trust in the transformative power of yoga to guide me on my journey.

This mission statement is not set in stone. As you evolve, it should too, reflecting your growth and serving as a constant reminder of your commitment to the yoga journey. Crafting this statement is a mindful exercise that instills clarity, direction, and purpose into your yoga practice. Let it light your path.

Guided Meditation: A Celebration of Your Inner Light

Meditation is a remarkable tool that can aid us in reconnecting with our inner selves. Today, we will engage in a special journey, a celebration of your inner light.

How to Engage with the Guided Meditation

Before we begin, make sure to find a quiet, peaceful space where you won't be disturbed. Sit comfortably, close your eyes, and take a few deep, cleansing breaths. Be open and receptive, and remember that there's no "right" or "wrong" way to meditate.

A Journey Within

Begin by visualizing a warm, radiant light at your core. It's your inner light, your unique spark. Feel it pulsing, vibrating with life, with your essence. It's beautiful, radiant, and full of boundless potential.

Now, let the light expand within you, filling every cell of your body, every corner of your being. As it expands, let it wash away any darkness, any stress, any tension that you may be holding onto. As it cleanses you, feel yourself becoming lighter, brighter, and more vibrant.

Picture this light expanding outwards, beyond your physical body, filling the room around you. This is your energy field, your aura. It is pure, it is powerful, and it's a beacon of positivity and strength.

Imagine your light touching those around you, affecting their lives positively. Feel the joy, the satisfaction that comes from making a difference, from making the world a brighter place with your unique light.

Finally, express gratitude for your inner light, for the positivity it brings into your life, for the difference it makes in the world.

Reflection Journal: Documenting Your Experience

After your meditation, take a moment to reflect and write about your experience.

1. How did the meditation make you feel?
2. What emotions did your inner light stir within you?

3. How can you use your inner light to make a positive difference in your world?

Reflecting on these questions will deepen your connection with your inner light and help you understand its transformative potential. As you write, remember, your inner light is a beacon of hope, strength, and positivity, capable of influencing not only your life but also those around you. Let's celebrate it every day!

Final Thoughts: Continuing Your Yoga Adventure with Confidence and Joy

Stepping Forward with Joy and Confidence

As we near the end of this book, it's important to recognize that your yoga adventure is only just beginning. Throughout these pages, you've embarked on a transformational journey, learning and growing along the way. But remember, yoga is a lifelong practice. It's about cultivating inner peace, resilience, and joy - qualities that will serve you well in all facets of your life.

In the spirit of celebrating your journey, let's revisit Tina's transformation. From a single mother overwhelmed by life's demands to a woman finding balance through Hatha Yoga and Ashtanga. Her journey echoes the potential of your own. It's proof that with patience, perseverance, and an open heart, you can manifest a deeper connection with your inner self, resulting in an empowered and fulfilling life.

Anecdote: The Unfolding Journey of Yoga

Consider Dylan, a military veteran who grappled with PTSD. Yoga became his lifeline, his path to healing. And it wasn't just about the physical practice, but the community he found - a network of fellow veterans on similar journeys, proving that healing can be a collective endeavor. It showed him that yoga isn't a destination but a continuous journey of self-discovery, healing, and growth. His story serves as an inspiration, reminding us that, with yoga, we're never alone.

Your Personal Action Plan

Now it's your turn. It's time to sketch out the next steps of your yoga adventure. Here's a simple action plan template to get you started:

Goal Setting: What do you wish to achieve through your continued yoga practice? More strength? Better flexibility? Inner peace? Write down your goals.

_____
_____
_____

Dedicated Practice: How often will you practice? Will it be daily, every other day, or twice a week? What time of day works best for you?

_____
_____
_____

Exploration: What styles of yoga would you like to explore next? Are there any workshops or retreats you would like to attend?

_____
_____
_____

Community Engagement: How will you engage with the yoga community? Will you join a local studio, participate in online forums, or share your journey on social media?

_____
_____
_____

Reflection: Reflect on your journey every week. How are you progressing towards your goals? What challenges are you facing, and how can you overcome them?

_____
_____
_____

Use this plan to chart your path forward, adapting it as your needs and goals evolve. Your yoga journey, like life, will have its ups and downs. There will be moments of revelation and times of struggle. But remember, the essence of yoga is patience and self-love. Embrace your practice with joy and confidence, and remember to celebrate the unique inner light within you.

As you continue on your yoga journey, carry the spirit of this book with you - the stories, the insights, the meditations - as a guide. Embrace the practice with an open heart, remain curious, and most importantly, never forget to honor and celebrate your inner light. Happy yoga adventuring!

The Journey of Self-Discovery and Transformation

As we close this chapter, we must remind ourselves of the incredible journey we've embarked on. Yoga, in its deepest sense, is a profound journey of self-discovery and transformation, a lifelong expedition that grows richer, deeper, and more fulfilling with each step.

A Transformative Tale: Embracing Change Through Yoga

Consider the story of Serenity, a yoga practitioner whose life was deeply altered by her yoga journey. When Serenity first stepped onto her yoga mat, she saw it as merely a way to improve her physical fitness. Over time, she noticed changes that went far beyond her physical body. She felt a newfound peace within herself, a profound sense of inner strength and clarity that helped her navigate through life's challenges with grace. This transformation continues to inspire her each day, strengthening her resolve to delve deeper into the world of yoga.

Your Inner Wisdom Vision Board

Now, let's create your Inner Wisdom Vision Board. On a blank canvas, envision and note down your dreams, desires, and goals in your yoga journey. Draw images or write words that resonate with your yogic aspirations. Place it somewhere you'll see daily to inspire you as you continue your journey.

Final Reflections and Actions

Reflect on this journey, ponder upon what you've learned, and consider how these teachings have altered your perceptions and behavior. Have you noticed any changes in yourself, however subtle they might be? As your next step, I challenge you to take one yoga principle we've discussed and consciously apply it in your daily life for the next week.

As we conclude this chapter, it's vital to remember that yoga is more than a practice; it's a lifelong adventure of exploration and transformation. Every breath, every pose, every moment of mindfulness is a step forward in this exciting journey.

Looking Ahead

As you continue to delve deeper into the world of yoga, remember that yoga is not confined to your mat - it's a lifestyle. In our next journey together, we'll explore integrating yoga principles into everyday life. As the saying goes, "Yoga is not about touching your toes, it's about what you learn on the way down." Keep that curiosity and eagerness to learn as we venture forth in this journey of self-discovery and transformation. Namaste.

21

Yoga as a Lifestyle: Integrating Yoga Principles into Everyday Life

We have traversed a remarkable path together, embarking on an enriching journey through the transformative world of yoga. Remember Serenity's story, a testament to yoga's transformative power? Like her, you too have been on a journey of self-discovery and transformation. You've seen glimpses of how yoga transcends the physical and imbues every facet of life with grace, resilience, and profound serenity.

Exploring Yoga: Beyond Physical Postures

In the words of the ancient sage, Patanjali, "Yoga is the stilling of the changing states of the mind." This is where the true essence of yoga lies - not in the flexibility of our bodies, but the resilience of our minds, the compassion in our hearts, the radiance of our souls.

It's time to unfurl the mat of your everyday life, to infuse every moment, every breath with the principles of yoga. Yoga, at its core, is a lifestyle, a radiant, resolute way of living that calls for authenticity, courage, and boundless love. It's not just about touching your toes but about what you learn on the journey down.

Are You Living Yoga?

Let's begin this final chapter of our shared adventure by gauging how much you've already integrated the yogic philosophy into your life. Let's delve into a little self-reflection together. Ready for a brief, enlightening quiz? a mirror that reflects your current journey.

No judgments, no expectations - simply a chance to witness where you stand now and where you might want to steer your path.

Quiz: Your Yogic Lifestyle

1. Can you recall a recent situation where you consciously practiced mindfulness? How did it make you feel?
2. Do you apply the concept of 'Ahimsa' (non-harming) in your interactions with others and yourself?
3. How well do you manage stress and challenges with a balanced, peaceful mind?
4. Are you living authentically, aligning your actions with your values and inner truth?
5. How often do you practice gratitude and cultivate joy in your everyday life?

Reflect on your responses, not as final verdicts, but as signposts pointing towards the next phase of your journey. Remember, there are no 'good' or 'bad' answers - only truthful ones. This quiz is merely a tool to illuminate your path, a compass guiding your steps towards a lifestyle imbued with love, shine, and the spirit of 'No F*cks to Give'.

Welcome, dear reader, to this final stage of our shared exploration, where we'll weave the philosophy of yoga into the fabric of your everyday life, truly embracing 'Love, Shine, and No F*cks to Give'.

The Importance of Living Yoga Off the Mat

In our penultimate chapter, we touched upon the transformative power of yoga and its ability to permeate our everyday lives. Now, as we move towards the end of our journey together, let's delve deeper into this concept. Yoga is not just an exercise routine, a series of postures, or a meditative practice; it is a way of life.

Yoga teaches us that we are far more than just our physical bodies. It is a holistic approach to wellness that nurtures the mind, body, and spirit in equal measure. Integrating yoga principles into daily life means extending these teachings beyond the mat. Yoga encourages us to practice mindfulness, compassion, gratitude, and kindness, not just during our practice but throughout the day. This integration allows us to experience a deeper connection with ourselves, others, and the world around us.

Living Yoga in Practice: Angela's Story

Consider, for example, Angela, a graduate student who incorporated box breathing to cope with academic stress. The benefits she derived didn't stop at her yoga mat's edge. Instead, they filtered into her study patterns, her interactions with colleagues, and her approach to stressors. Her yoga journey was not confined to her mat; it transformed her life.

Reflection: Living Yoga Off the Mat

Reflect on your own experience with yoga. How have the lessons from your practice influenced your daily life? Do you find yourself more mindful of your breath when under stress? Are you more aware of your body's needs and signals? How has yoga influenced your interactions with others?

Consider ways you could further embody your yoga practice in daily life. Maybe it's taking a few moments each day to ground yourself with a deep breath. Perhaps it's showing more compassion to yourself and others. Or maybe it's cultivating gratitude each day. The possibilities are endless.

Quiz: Assessing Your Integration of Yoga Principles

Let's take a moment to assess how well you're incorporating yoga principles into your daily life. Consider the following questions:

1. Do you bring mindfulness to your daily tasks?
2. Do you practice gratitude regularly?
3. Are you making conscious choices in line with yogic principles?
4. Are you using breathwork techniques during moments of stress?
5. Are you bringing a sense of compassion and kindness into your interactions with others?

By living yoga off the mat, we invite a deeper sense of balance, peace, and wellness into our lives. As we close this chapter and this book, remember that the journey doesn't end here. Like a pose held and deepened, your yoga practice is something to grow and develop, breathing life into every moment, on and off the mat. Namaste.

Applying Yogic Principles to Relationships, Work, and Daily Activities

As we draw towards the end of this enlightening journey, it's time to revisit and refresh our understanding of the essential teachings: bringing yogic philosophy into our daily life. Let's recap how yoga, far beyond the mat, can invigorate our relationships, our work, and our everyday tasks.

Revisiting Yoga in Relationships

Our relationships are a reflection of the dance between our inner selves and the world. Remember how we spoke about empathy in our interactions, a principle borrowed from our yoga practice. It's about truly understanding others, just as we've learned to understand our bodies' needs and responses during yoga.

The importance of patience and compassion cannot be overstated. In our yoga practice, we never force a pose; we allow it to develop naturally. This approach, if applied to our relationships, can pave the way for more meaningful connections.

Finally, remember the power of Satya, honesty, in our relationships. Just as we maintain an honest relationship with our bodies and minds during our yoga practice, we should strive to do the same with our loved ones.

Re-emphasizing Yogic Principles at Work

Our professional life can also benefit immensely from the application of yogic principles. James, a software developer, used to struggle with deadlines and the unending stress they brought. When he began to incorporate mindfulness, a cornerstone of yoga, into his day, he noticed a shift. He was able to concentrate better, his decision-making improved, and he managed his time more effectively. It transformed not just his work, but his overall sense of well-being.. When we give our complete attention to each task, just as we do to each breath during our practice, we can enhance our productivity and make our work more enjoyable.

Let's also remember Aparigraha, the practice of non-attachment, which teaches us to value the journey over the destination. In our careers, this could mean finding joy in our work itself, rather than being solely focused on the outcomes.

Lastly, recall the essence of Sangha, our yoga community, and how fostering such a sense of support and togetherness in the workplace can lead to a more harmonious environment.

Yoga in Daily Activities: A Recap

Yogic principles can breathe new life into even the most mundane activities. From cooking with mindfulness to expressing gratitude at mealtimes, and even approaching cleaning as a form of energy-clearing asana, we've explored numerous ways to infuse our day with yoga.

A Reflective Recap

To further consolidate our learning, let's reflect on these principles. Write down your answers to these questions:

1. How have you managed to cultivate more empathy, patience, compassion, and honesty in your relationships through yoga?
2. In what ways have the principles of yoga improved your work-life balance and job satisfaction?
3. How have your daily routines been transformed by integrating mindfulness or gratitude?

As we close this chapter and the book, remember that yoga is more than just asanas; it's a way of life. Continue incorporating these principles into every area of your life. Don't forget, it's a journey—be gentle with yourself as you continue to evolve.

Practicing Mindfulness, Gratitude, and Compassion in Everyday Life

As we continue the final chapter of our journey together, let's delve deeper into the heart of a yogic lifestyle, which thrives on the bedrock of mindfulness, gratitude, and compassion.

Embracing Mindfulness, Gratitude, and Compassion

Mindfulness, the gentle act of being present and fully engaged with the here and now, is a virtue we've consistently practiced on our mats. Taking this principle off the mat, it's about savoring our morning coffee, truly listening when a friend speaks, or feeling the breeze on a casual stroll.

Gratitude, another essential yogic principle, invites us to cherish and acknowledge the blessings in our lives, both big and small. Like the constant cycle of inhalation and exhalation in our practice, gratitude effortlessly flows into our daily life, nourishing our hearts with joy and contentment.

Lastly, compassion is the loving-kindness we extend not only to others but also to ourselves. As our yoga practice teaches us to respect our bodies' limits, compassion guides us to understand and empathize with others' struggles.

One simple practice you can adopt is to spend five minutes each morning on mindful breathing. Sit comfortably, close your eyes, and focus your attention on your breath. Notice the sensation of the air entering and leaving your body. When your mind wanders, gently bring your attention back to your breath. Starting your day with mindfulness can set the tone for the rest of your day.

Practical Tip: Cultivating These Practices

To weave mindfulness into your everyday life, start small. For instance, dedicate your first five waking minutes to mindfulness, observing your surroundings, feelings, and thoughts without judgment.

For gratitude, keep a 'blessings jar,' where each day, you write a note about something you're grateful for and put it in the jar. On tough days, pull out a note to remind yourself of your blessings.

To cultivate compassion, practice metta, or loving-kindness meditation. Repeat phrases like "May I be safe. May I be happy. May I be healthy. May I live with ease," and gradually extend these wishes to others.

Date: _____

Mindfulness

Today's Mindful Moment: _____

Observations/Insights: _____

Gratitude

Today's Blessing(s): _____

Feeling of Gratitude (On a scale of 1-10): ____

Compassion

Acts of Compassion (For self/others): _____

Reflections/Feelings: _____

Keeping a journal encourages consistency and allows you to look back on your progress. Even on days where these practices may feel challenging, remember, it's your journey, and every step, no matter how small, is progress.

As we continue to explore the application of these principles, remember that they aren't just actions but rather a mindset that seeps into every aspect of our lives. As you continue your journey beyond this book, may your path be enriched with the joy and fulfillment these practices bring.

Navigating Life's Challenges with a Yogic Mindset

A yogic mindset is much like a compass, providing direction amidst life's tempests. It does not necessarily change the storm around us, but it can drastically alter our experience of it. It's about finding equilibrium and resilience in an often tumultuous world.

Embracing the Yogic Mindset amidst Challenges

The tools we cultivate through yoga – mindfulness, presence, gratitude, and compassion – are not confined to the four corners of our mats. Rather, they permeate into every aspect of our lives, helping us navigate personal trials with grace and fortitude.

Consider Emma's journey. A high-pressure lifestyle had left her feeling spent, both physically and emotionally. But as she embraced pranayama, a method of conscious breath control, she found a renewed sense of balance. She began experiencing deeper connections with her body, mind, and spirit, transforming the way she interacted with the world and faced its challenges.

Each obstacle we encounter can be seen as a kind of yoga pose – demanding balance, strength, and a gentle approach. Just as we adjust our bodies in asana practice to find comfort and steadiness, a yogic mindset can help us adjust our perspectives towards life's hurdles, enabling us to handle them with more resilience and serenity.

Personal Story: James's Triumph Over Life's Marathon

Take James, a marathon runner who faced an unexpected injury. The prospect of not being able to run – his true passion – was devastating. However, in his physical rehabilitation, he was introduced to Yin Yoga, a practice that emphasizes deep release and patience. Initially, James struggled with the slow pace and stillness. But as he stuck with it, he found a deep sense of release physically and mentally. Yin taught him to embrace the slow process of healing, offering lessons in resilience that he could carry off the mat.

This experience didn't eliminate his obstacles. Instead, it transformed how he perceived his situation. He adopted a mindset that allowed him to understand that healing, much like running a marathon, requires patience, endurance, and a gentle approach with oneself.

Reflecting on Your Yogic Journey

Now, let's take a moment to apply this mindset to your own life. Reflect on the following questions:

1. What is a personal challenge that you're currently facing?
2. How might you apply the principles of yoga – presence, acceptance, and compassion – to this situation?
3. Are there specific yoga practices that could support you in this situation? (e.g., a calming pranayama practice for stress, or a grounding meditation for feelings of instability)

Remember, just as each yoga pose requires gentle, patient adjustment, so too does our approach to life's challenges. Embrace the journey. Find strength in the struggle. And above all, remember to breathe. As you navigate through your own life's marathon, may the principles of yoga guide you towards balance, resilience, and a harmonious perspective.

Embracing the Yamas and Niyamas in Daily Life

As we reach the culmination of our journey together, let's continue our exploration of the yamas and niyamas, the moral and ethical guidelines of yoga, as we learn to truly embrace them in our daily life. While understanding their conceptual essence is key, their real power lies in the integration into our day-to-day existence. Let's dive deep into these precious pearls of wisdom and start practicing them, not just on the yoga mat, but in the bigger arena of life.

Living the Yamas and Niyamas

Each day presents numerous opportunities to live the yamas and niyamas. Whether it's responding with patience and compassion to a frustrating situation (Ahimsa), or finding satisfaction in simple pleasures instead of constant consumption (Aparigraha), every moment is a chance to practice these principles.

Likewise, the niyamas offer an internal compass guiding our personal growth. Cultivating discipline (Tapas) might involve maintaining a daily meditation practice, while studying and understanding ourselves (Svadhyaya) could be as simple as reflecting on our reactions to daily events.

Practical Tip: Everyday Actions, Extraordinary Transformation

Begin by choosing one yama or niyama to focus on each week. Reflect upon it in the morning, reminding yourself of its essence. Throughout the day, actively look for situations to practice this principle.

For instance, during a week focusing on Satya, consciously observe your conversations. Are you fully expressing your truth? Or are you holding back or modifying to avoid conflict or discomfort? Remember, it's about truthful expression that also embodies Ahimsa – kindness and non-harm.

Similarly, a week of Santosha might involve starting each day by writing down three things you're grateful for, and then striving to find contentment in your day as it unfolds, without chasing after external validation or craving for more.

Your Daily Yamas and Niyamas Checklist

Create a daily checklist for your chosen yama or niyama. As you progress through the day, reflect on and note the moments when you consciously practiced the principle. Don't be discouraged if you forget or falter; the journey is about awareness and growth, not perfection. Just as in yoga practice, some days we stand firm in our asanas, some days we wobble. And that's perfectly okay.

Daily Yamas and Niyamas Practice Checklist

Date: _____

Chosen Yama/Niyama for the Week: _____

Morning Reflection:

- **Principle Understanding:** Briefly jot down your understanding of the chosen Yama/Niyama. This will serve as your intention for the day.
  _____
  _____
  _____

- **Anticipated Opportunities:** Can you anticipate any situations today where you could practice your chosen Yama/Niyama? Describe them
  _____
  _____
  _____

Midday Reflection:

- **Observations:** Have you noticed any situations so far today where you could (or did) apply your chosen Yama/Niyama?
  _____
  _____
  _____

- **Challenges:** Did you face any challenges in practicing your Yama/Niyama? How did you respond to these challenges?
  _____
  _____
  _____

Evening Reflection:

- **Successes:** Write down instances where you successfully practiced your Yama/Niyama today.
  _____
  _____
  _____

- **Challenges:** Were there any moments you forgot or faltered in practicing your chosen principle? How can you approach this differently tomorrow?

  _____
  _____
  _____

- **Feelings and Thoughts:** Reflect on how you feel about your progress. What thoughts or feelings arose during the practice of this Yama/Niyama today?

  _____
  _____
  _____

Remember, it's not about how many times you faltered, but about how many times you noticed, adjusted, and continued your practice. Your journey towards integrating the Yamas and Niyamas into your daily life is one of progress and patience. Keep going!

Embracing the Journey

Remember, incorporating yamas and niyamas into your daily life isn't about strict adherence to rules, but rather about understanding their essence and applying them in ways that resonate with your own unique life. They are not rigid commandments but flexible guidelines to support us on our journey toward self-realization. They remind us that yoga isn't confined to the mat or the studio but is a holistic practice that weaves into the fabric of our everyday lives.

Through this exploration and practice of the yamas and niyamas, you're not just learning ancient principles, but truly living them. The transformation might not happen overnight, and that's okay. Even a small step towards Ahimsa, a minute dedicated to Santosha, or an attempt to embrace Aparigraha is a victory to celebrate.

Remember, this journey is not a destination but a path – a path of awakening, understanding, and unfolding. So, dear reader, as we conclude this book, let's remember the essence of Ishvara Pranidhana, the final niyama – surrender. Trust the journey, surrender to the process, and see how the yamas and niyamas beautifully unfold and weave into the tapestry of your life.

Reflect for a moment on the journey we've taken together. Remember in the earlier chapters, when we spoke about the first time stepping on a yoga mat and feeling that incredible connection of mind, body, and spirit? That was the first step, and look at how far you've come.

Recall the stories we've shared throughout this book. The struggles, the triumphs, the moments of clarity - they've all led to this point, to a deeper understanding of yoga and self.

Interactive Exercise: Reflecting on Your Personal Yoga Journey and Setting Intentions for the Future

The beautiful journey of yoga is deeply personal, ever-evolving, and eternally enlightening. Each of us embarks on this path at our own pace, guided by our unique experiences, challenges, and aspirations. This exercise invites you to pause, look back at your journey, and set powerful intentions for the future.

Reflecting on Your Yoga Journey

Reflecting on your yoga journey isn't about judging or rating your practice but rather about understanding how far you've come and the transformation you've undergone.

> **Step 1:** Start with recalling your initial days. What led you to yoga? What were your initial challenges and victories?
>
> **Step 2:** Move onto significant milestones. Have there been any 'aha' moments? Did yoga help you through a challenging period?
>
> **Step 3:** Think about the present. How has your understanding of yoga deepened? Has your practice shifted or evolved?

Setting Future Intentions

Setting intentions provides a guiding light for your yoga journey, helping you stay focused and grounded.

- **Step 1:** Reflect on what you seek from your future yoga practice. It could be anything from developing a daily meditation habit to embracing a particular Yama or Niyama.
- **Step 2:** Ensure your intention is realistic and resonates with you deeply. Setting an intention is like planting a seed. Nurture it with consistent practice.

- **Step 3:** Visualize yourself fulfilling this intention. How would it feel? Visualization can strengthen your resolve and motivation.

Reflective Template:

Use this simple template to document your reflections and intentions.

Date: _____

Past Reflections

My Yoga Beginnings:

1. Why I started yoga:
   _____
   _____
   _____

2. Initial challenges and victories:
   _____
   _____
   _____

Significant Milestones:

1. 'Aha' moments:
   _____
   _____
   _____

2. How yoga supported me during challenging times:
   _____
   _____
   _____

Present Reflections:

1. How my understanding of yoga has deepened:
   _____
   _____
   _____

2. How my practice has evolved:
   _____
   _____
   _____

Future Intentions

1. What I seek from my future yoga practice:
   _____
   _____
   _____

2. Why this intention resonates with me:
   _____
   _____
   _____

3. How I visualize myself fulfilling this intention:
   _____
   _____
   _____

Remember, your yoga journey is unique, just like you. Embrace its twists and turns, its peaks and valleys. In this dance of self-discovery, every step you take brings you closer to your true self. Enjoy the journey. Namaste.

Guided Meditation: Envisioning Your Ideal Yogic Lifestyle

Embarking on the yogic journey, we cultivate a sacred bond with our bodies, minds, and spirits. We practice, breathe, and grow – but often, we forget to dream. This final chapter invites you to dream and to visualize your ideal yogic lifestyle. Let's do this through a guided meditation.

Embarking on a Guided Meditation

Guided meditation helps us focus our minds and set intentions. It's like having a personal guide for our mental journey. Here's how to engage effectively:

- **Tip 1:** Choose a quiet, peaceful space and a comfortable position.
- **Tip 2:** Let go of any expectations. Embrace the journey and trust where your mind leads you.
- **Tip 3:** After the meditation, take a moment to dwell in that space of peace and tranquility.

A Guided Journey to Your Ideal Yogic Lifestyle

Close your eyes and take a deep, nourishing breath. Picture a ball of light at the center of your heart, radiating peace and serenity. With every breath, this light grows, until it envelops you completely.

In this space of peace, imagine stepping onto a path. This is the path of your ideal yogic lifestyle. What does it look like? Is it nestled in the hustle and bustle of a city or in the tranquil expanse of nature?

As you walk this path, you come across your ideal daily routine. What does your yoga practice look like? How does your day unfold? Notice the food you eat, the books you read, the way you work, and the way you rest.

Now, envision yourself walking this path every day, immersing yourself in this ideal lifestyle. Notice how it feels in your body, mind, and spirit. Take a moment to soak it all in.

Reflecting on the Journey: A Final Journal Exercise

Now that you've envisioned your ideal yogic lifestyle, it's time to document it in your journal. You've grown proficient with your journal over this journey, and it's time to use this tool to crystallize your vision.

Here are some reflection prompts:

- **My Ideal Yogic Lifestyle:** Describe the path you saw in your meditation. What did it look like? Feel like?

- **My Ideal Daily Routine:** Detail your perfect day, including your yoga practice, meals, work, and rest.
- **Steps Toward My Ideal Lifestyle:** Identify small, achievable steps you can take towards your envisioned lifestyle.
- **Feelings and Insights:** Write down any feelings or insights that arose during the meditation.

Remember, like your yoga journey, your ideal lifestyle is a vision unique to you. Embrace it, strive for it, and allow it to evolve with you. As we close this chapter and this book, remember that every end is a new beginning, a step closer to your true self. Namaste.

Final Thoughts: Continuing Your Yoga Adventure with Confidence, Joy, and Inner Light

It's been an extraordinary journey we've embarked on, from the first page where we opened the door to the world of 'Love, Shine, and No F*cks to Give', to this point where we stand, poised and ready to integrate yoga principles into every aspect of our lives.

Think back to the beginning of our journey, when we first explored the concept of 'Love, Shine, and No F*cks to Give'. How have those ideas manifested in your life? Remember the stories of personal transformation that we discussed - now you're part of that legacy too.

Reflect on the yogic mindset that you've embraced, the transformation you've felt in your body, your heart, your very spirit. From these experiences, draw strength and confidence to continue this adventure of self-love, radiant happiness, and unabashed authenticity that yoga offers.

In the spirit of 'No F*cks to Give', it's now your moment to embody your unique truth and shine brightly without inhibition. Let's remember the story of Serenity - how she grew stronger and more vibrant with each yoga practice, with each conscious breath. Take her story as your inspiration, infuse your life with the light of love and courage.

Your Next Steps: Embracing the Lifestyle of 'Love, Shine, and No F*cks to Give'

As a closing interactive element, pull out your Inner Wisdom Vision Board. Reflect on the goals you've set for yourself, the dreams you've decided to chase. As we step into this new stage of our yoga journey, decide which yoga principles you'll integrate into your daily life this week.

Consider the daily challenges you face - how can the mindset of 'No F*cks to Give' transform these experiences? Challenge yourself to approach your life with the radical authenticity that we've explored. Consider this your call to action.

Conclusion: Yoga as a Lifestyle

Embrace the lifestyle of 'Love, Shine, and No Fcks to Give', and remember that yoga is more than the poses - it's a beacon that lights up the path to our most authentic selves. It guides us to live boldly, love fiercely, shine brightly, and to give no unnecessary f*cks along the way. With every breath and every pose, let's choose love, let's choose to shine, and let's choose to give no f*cks that do not serve our growth.

Although we've reached the end of this book, remember that the true journey continues off the mat and into the world. This book may conclude here, but your story of 'Love, Shine, and No F*cks to Give' is just beginning. Keep exploring, keep shining, and keep being unapologetically you. Namaste.

About the Author

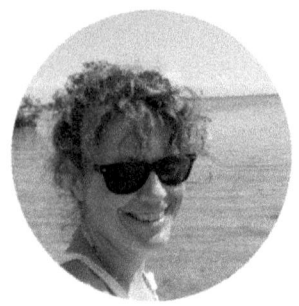

S.G. Bloomfield, a versatile author and registered yoga instructor since 2017, brings a unique perspective to her work, combining her passion for yoga, mindfulness, and creativity. Born and raised in Canada, S.G. Bloomfield has traveled extensively to both well-known and off-the-beaten-path locations, immersing herself in diverse cultures and experiences. Her adventures have not only inspired her writing but also fueled her artistic pursuits as the owner, designer, and artist behind Home Time Art, an Etsy shop specializing in modern, minimalist, and spiritual high-quality printable art.

S.G. Bloomfield's writing style is a blend of personal, instructional, and narrative elements, characterized by its conversational, informative, and imaginative voice. Her ability to connect with readers stems from her own experiences teaching yoga, including unique classes such as Kid Yoga and Puppy Yoga. She has also hosted popular Wine and Paint parties and Paint Night events for all ages.

In addition to her adult non-fiction yoga guidebooks, S.G. Bloomfield is also the author of the delightful Little Yogi series of children's illustration books. Through her diverse body of work, S.G. Bloomfield seeks to share the transformative power of yoga, mindfulness, and art with people of all ages and walks of life.

When she's not writing, teaching, or creating art, S.G. Bloomfield continues to explore the world and find new inspiration for her many endeavors. If you'd like to connect or learn more about her work, S.G. Bloomfield invites you to reach out and share your thoughts.

With Gratitude: A Message to My Readers

Thank you, dear reader, for joining me on this journey into the world of yoga, self-love, and inner peace. Writing "Love, Shine, and No F*cks to Give: A Guide to Embracing Your Inner Light through Yoga" has been an incredible journey of self-discovery and transformation.

In sharing my personal experiences, learnings, and the teachings from the sacred practice of yoga, my hope is that you find solace, strength, and an ignited spark within you to seek your own path of inner love and illumination. The stories, the instructions, the love, and the light that fill these pages are meant to serve as a beacon guiding you towards your innermost self.

I feel incredibly grateful for the One Love One Heart Yoga Studio in Beeton, Ontario, Canada, where my journey with yoga began. I dedicate this book to this sacred space and the extraordinary community it nurtures, for it is here that I discovered the transformative power of yoga.

But, my dear reader, this journey is far from over. It is just the beginning, and I can't wait to hear about your own experiences and transformations. I warmly welcome your insights, reflections, and stories.

If you have a few moments, I would truly appreciate it if you could leave a review for the book. Your thoughts and feedback not only help me grow as a writer but also help other readers discover this book. Remember, your voice matters - it can inspire and guide others on their journeys too.

Thank you once again for embracing this guide and embarking on this transformative journey with me. May your journey of self-love and self-discovery through yoga lead you to a life filled with authenticity, love, and an abundance of No F*cks to Give!

With Gratitude and Love,

S.G. Bloomfield

www.ingramcontent.com/pod-product-compliance
Lightning Source LLC
Chambersburg PA
CBHW042023100526
44587CB00029B/4278